P9-AOL-208

# Pediatric Splinting

## Selection, Fabrication, and Clinical Application of Upper Extremity Splints

**Laura Hogan,** OTR, BCP

**Tracey Uditsky,** OTR, BCP

Photographs by Jon N. Uditsky

**Therapy Skill Builders**®
a division of
The Psychological Corporation

555 Academic Court
San Antonio, Texas 78204-2498
1-800-228-0752

## Reproducing Pages from This Book

As described below, some of the pages in this book may be reproduced for instructional use (not for resale). To protect your book, make a photocopy of each reproducible page. Then use that copy as a master for photocopying.

Copyright © 1998 by

**Therapy
Skill Builders®**
a division of
The Psychological Corporation

555 Academic Court
San Antonio, Texas 78204-2498
1-800-228-0752

All rights reserved. No part of this publication may be
reproduced or transmitted in any form or by any means,
electronic or mechanical, including photocopy, recording,
or any information storage and retrieval system, without
permission in writing from the publisher.

Permission is hereby granted to reproduce the patterns
in this publication in complete pages, with the copyright
notice, for instructional use and not for resale.

*The Learning Curve Design* and *Therapy Skill Builders*
are registered trademarks of The Psychological Corporation.

Printed in the United States of America.

0761615148

3 4 5 6 7 8 9 10 11 12 A B C D E

## About the Authors

**Tracey Uditsky, OTR, BCP,** graduated from Loma Linda University in 1986 with a bachelor of arts degree in occupational therapy. She has 12 years of experience working with children in the San Bernardino County and Los Angeles County California Children Services programs. Tracey is self-employed as a pediatric OT consultant. She treats and consults with the regional center, CCS, and a local intervention program. She has written several articles on OT practice in pediatrics and has made numerous presentations to therapists, OT students, parents, and community agencies. She is an honorary clinical faculty member at both Loma Linda University and the University of Southern California. She received her AOTA Board Certification in Pediatrics in 1992.

**Laura Hogan, OTR, BCP,** earned her bachelor of science degree in occupational therapy in 1984 from Western Michigan University. For the past 14 years, she has been working in the field of pediatrics in a variety of settings, including NICU, acute inpatient, in-home health services and outpatient clinics. Currently, Laura is self-employed as a pediatric OT consultant. In 1988, she received her 8-week pediatric certification in neurodevelopmental treatment. She has previously lectured on a variety of pediatric topics and has written for several professional therapy publications. She received her AOTA Board Certification in Pediatrics in 1997.

# Contents

## Chapter **3**   Practical Tips for Fabrication and Wear ...............51

Chapter **4** **Splint Patterns and Fabrication Directions** ............................ 79

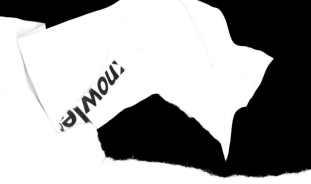

# Preface

With almost 25 years of combined experience in pediatrics, hundreds of splints under our belts, and countless lunch conversations about the new products we saw in catalogs, we still love to splint! We are happy to report that most of our splints are very successful, but, to be honest, they weren't always.

Before we started this book-writing endeavor, our goal was simply to locate some current, practical information on pediatric splinting. In our occupational therapy practices, which include teaching and consulting on numerous pediatric topics (including splinting), we labored to provide current, accurate information to our peers and colleagues. As we attempted to locate more references on pediatric splinting, we encountered the same frustration over and again: There just isn't a lot of information published on pediatric splinting. Although we did find some literature from those we like to call "the pediatric splinting pioneers"—Joyce MacKinnon, Charlotte Exner, and Janet Reymann—we were surprised that there were no existing textbooks to meet the needs of therapists on this broad and somewhat difficult topic.

Feeling the need to fill a gap in our profession, we combined our stacks of articles, patterns, and lecture notes and developed this manual, which we believe is practical and helpful for those clinicians who work with infants, children, and adults who have developmental disabilities. Although much of the information you will find herein is experimental, we have combined it with our personal experiences and information from the pioneers, adult splinting literature, and other various articles and sections of textbooks that include pediatric splints.

The splints that are presented are all splints with which we have had personal experience and success for our clients. The patterns included are our preferred patterns but there are others, and there are many variations of these patterns that you may know or prefer. After reading the text, we hope that you will feel more confident in your clinical decisions and free to customize your splints and try new ideas and materials. Adjust the patterns we have provided if you have the need; make them work for your patients. We encourage you to be creative and experiment. Our hope is that we have shared something that will make your therapeutic interventions a little more successful and a little easier. Enjoy the book.

*Tracey Uditsky and Laura Hogan*

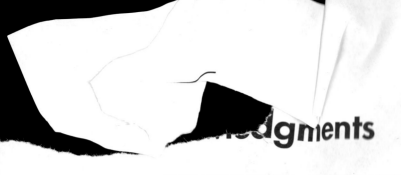

# Acknowledgments

This book was a collaborative effort. First of all we'd like to thank our husbands, Joe Reyes, Jr. and Jon Uditsky, for their endless patience and support, and for the absence of complaints regarding the roomfuls of splinting materials they have had to trip over since we started this endeavor. Jon was also our fabulous photographer. (If you had seen the pictures we had taken, you would be as grateful to him as we are.) Special thanks to Jessica Schuman and Cara Boucher for lending a helping hand. Last but not least, we would like to thank the occupational therapists from Los Angeles County California Children Services who, through their skills, creativity, clinical reasoning, and perseverance, have been a constant source of motivation for us. Without them, this book would not have been possible.

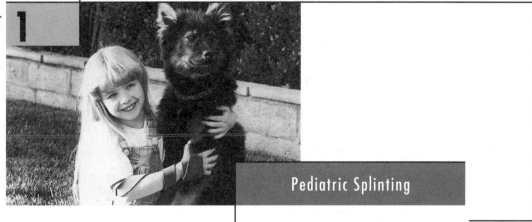

# Principles in Pediatric Splinting

Chapter **1**

Pediatric Splinting

## Introduction

Many consider pediatric splinting to be a specialty area. This is probably true. In every practice setting there are basic skills and advanced skills. Advanced skills in splinting usually are acquired through time, mentoring from others with more experience, advanced clinical training, and practice with clinical reasoning skills. Mastery is obtained after a thorough understanding of the pertinent basic information is developed.

For pediatric splinting, we define pertinent basic information as an understanding of the anatomy of the upper extremity; normal infant motor development, with emphasis on the development of the hand; and standard splinting design and fabrication principles.

In this chapter, you will review these three areas and learn more complex information related to pediatric splinting that will enable you to understand the advanced skills necessary to become proficient at splinting children. This includes how to assess thoroughly the upper extremity, prioritize problems, and identify goals for splinting. The chapter also contains information on selecting an appropriate splint based on identified problems and analyzing specific patient data to help you narrow your choices among the numerous variables in splinting, such as straps, dorsal versus volar splints, and material selection.

This chapter should serve as a reference when you are selecting splints and fabricating from the patterns and directions in Chapter 4.

## Anatomy of the Upper Extremity

To fabricate correct and effective upper extremity splints in any setting, a therapist must have a knowledge base in the anatomy and kinesiology of the arm and hand. It is beyond the scope and intent of this book to review in great detail the volumes of information written on anatomy and kinesiology of the upper extremity. The information provided here is intended for quick reference and review. However, thorough knowledge of the hand, with emphasis on bony structures and anatomical landmarks, will enable you to fabricate a variety of splints in the appropriate alignment that will be effective and comfortable to wear. A more thorough examination of upper extremity anatomy is recommended for any clinician who feels uncertain of basic anatomy and kinesiology. Please refer to the bibliography and Appendix A for resources on these topics.

## Anatomical Position and Motion

In order to define the components of the body and its movement patterns, we must begin with a description of standard anatomical body position. Anatomical position is defined as standing erect with the head, toes, and palms of the hands facing forward, the fingers extended (hand open), and the thumbs pointing away from the body (Figure 1.1). When the body is in this position, three imaginary planes are used to help describe body parts and their relationships with each other as movement occurs.

The frontal plane (also referred to as the coronal plane) is a vertical plane that divides the body into front and back parts. Motions that occur in this plane are defined as adduction (moving toward the middle of the body) and abduction (moving away from the middle of the body). At the wrist, adduction is referred to as ulnar deviation, and abduction is referred to as radial deviation.

The longitudinal plane (also referred to as the sagittal or mid-sagittal plane) is also a vertical plane. It divides the body into right and left parts. Motions that occur in this

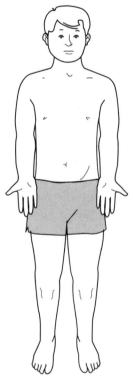

Figure **1.1** Standard anatomical body position

plane are defined as flexion, extension, and hyperextension. Flexion typically means decreasing the angle between two body segments, such as bending the arm at the elbow. It also is used to describe the motion when a body part goes forward. Extension typically means increasing the angle between two body segments, such as opening the arm at the elbow. Likewise, extension can describe the motion when a body part goes backward. Hyperextension is when the motion goes beyond the anatomical reference point.

The transverse plane (also referred to as the horizontal plane) divides the body into upper and lower parts. When the transverse plane intersects with the longitudinal plane, movement in the transverse plane is referred to as rotation. Rotation can be internal (toward the middle of the body) or external (toward the edges of the body). Internal rotation of the forearm is known as pronation, while external rotation of the forearm is known as supination.

After such a straightforward explanation of how adduction and abduction occur in the frontal plane, and flexion and extension occur in the longitudinal plane, we must point out that the thumb is considered a *special case* (Lehmkuhl and Smith, 1983). You will find that description of motions of the thumb varies among sources. To clarify this and to help you follow the splint fabrication directions in Chapter 4, in this text abduction and palmar abduction at the thumb refer to the same motion. Starting from standard anatomical position, abduction and adduction of the thumb occur in the longitudinal (sagittal) plane (Figure 1.2). Furthermore, extension and radial abduction of the thumb are often used interchangeably. Flexion of the thumb brings it into the palm. Extension places it back in anatomical position. Flexion and extension of the thumb occur in the frontal (coronal) plane (Figure 1.3).

In relation to anatomical position, there are a few other terms relevant to upper extremity splinting with which you will need to be familiar to understand the splint fabrication directions in Chapter 4. *Dorsal* refers to the back surface of the hand where the knuckles are located. *Volar* and *palmar* both refer to the concave surface of the hand where the pads of the fingers are located. The *ulnar* side of the hand is the side with the little finger. The *radial* side of the hand is the side with the thumb. The *lateral* side of the hand always indicates the radial side because the palm is up when the body is in anatomical position. *Proximal* and distal relate the location of one area or joint to another. Proximal refers to a point closer to the body and farther from the tips of the fingers. *Distal* is the opposite and

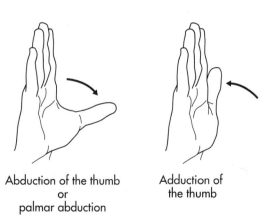

Abduction of the thumb
or
palmar abduction

Adduction of
the thumb

Figure **1.2**   Abduction and adduction of the thumb occurs in
the longitudinal plane

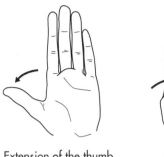

Extension of the thumb
or
radial abduction

Flexion of
the thumb

Figure **1.3** Extension and flexion of the thumb occurs in the
frontal plane

refers to a point closer to the fingertips and farther from the body. The fingers of the hand can easily be identified using index, middle, ring, and little. The digits of the hand often are numbered 1 to 5 to help identify them (the thumb being number 1, the little finger being number 5).

## Bones

The bones form the framework on which the rest of the body is built. They are held together by ligaments and tendons and moved by the muscles. The structures of bones are complex. Bones are comprised of osseous tissue and contain their own blood supply. Aside from the teeth, bones are the hardest structure in the body, yet they are slightly elastic and can withstand tension and compression to a remarkable degree (Clemente, 1985). Each upper extremity contains 32 bones (Figure 1.4).

The pectoral girdle, the upper limb, and the forearm are composed of five bones: the clavicle, scapula, humerus, radius, and ulna. There are eight carpal bones in the wrist. Four are proximal: the pisiform, lunate, scaphoid, and triquetrum. Four are distal: the hamate, capitate, trapezoid, and trapezium. The hand contains five metacarpal bones. The fingers and thumb contain 14 phalanges, five of which are proximal, four are middle (there is no middle phalange on the thumb), and five are distal.

## Joints

A joint is an articulation where the bones of the body meet and where movement occurs. The structure of a joint varies based on whether movement occurs and, if it does occur, on the type and degree of movement. The joints of the hand and arm are multiple and complex. A moveable joint is comprised of bones, a layer of cartilage that covers and provides a smooth surface at the end of the bones, a sheath of fibrous tissue known as the capsule, and a synovial membrane that lines the capsule and produces synovial fluid to lubricate the movements of the joint.

In addition, joints are stabilized and positioned by the muscles that pass over them. Moveable joints frequently are classified as gliding (found in the wrist), hinge (found in the fingers), and ball-and-socket (found at the shoulder). Joints of the wrist and hand and their common abbreviations are identified in Figure 1.5 on page 6.

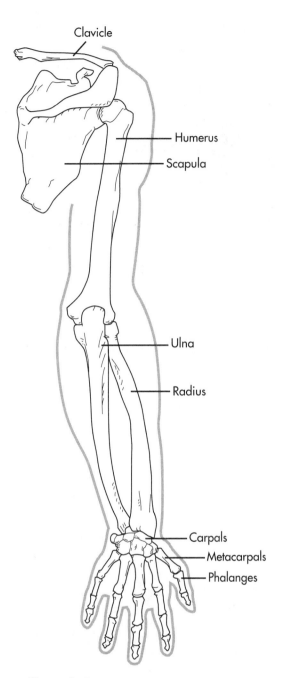

Clavicle

Humerus

Scapula

Ulna

Radius

Carpals

Metacarpals

Phalanges

Figure **1.4**   Bones of the upper extremity

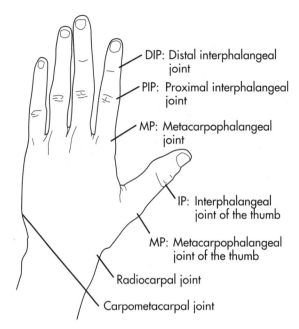

DIP: Distal interphalangeal joint

PIP: Proximal interphalangeal joint

MP: Metacarpophalangeal joint

IP: Interphalangeal joint of the thumb

MP: Metacarpophalangeal joint of the thumb

Radiocarpal joint

Carpometacarpal joint

Figure **1.5** Joints of the wrist and hand

## Muscles

There are numerous skeletal muscles in the arm and hand. Muscles are composed of tissues that originate and insert into bones via tendons. Muscles use energy to contract. The ability of muscle groups to contract and relax as they cross over a joint results in movement at that joint in the direction in which the muscle fibers lie.

The hand contains both intrinsic and extrinsic muscles. Intrinsic muscles are those whose origin and insertions are located distal to the wrist. Extrinsic muscles have origins proximal to the wrist and insertions distal to the wrist into the palm, thumb, or fingers. The muscle bellies of the extrinsic muscles are located in the forearm; the distal tendon of the extrinsic muscle crosses the carpals and inserts into the hand. The intrinsic and extrinsic muscles are innervated by the radial, ulnar, and median nerves.

Muscles of the upper extremity can be placed into eight main muscle groups: muscles acting on the scapula; muscles acting on the shoulder joint; flexors of the elbow joint; extensors of the elbow joint; flexors of the wrist, hand, and fingers; extensors of the wrist, hand, and fingers; forearm muscles acting on the thumb; and muscles of the hand (intrinsics only). The muscular system of the upper extremity is vast and complex. Figure 1.6 depicts the muscle groups.

## Connective Tissue

Although the bones of the arm offer the principle support in the upper extremity, the role of the connective tissue cannot be overlooked. Fascia is a three-dimensional web of connective tissue that runs in both the longitudinal and transverse planes without any origins or insertions. The primary function of connective tissue is to support posture and

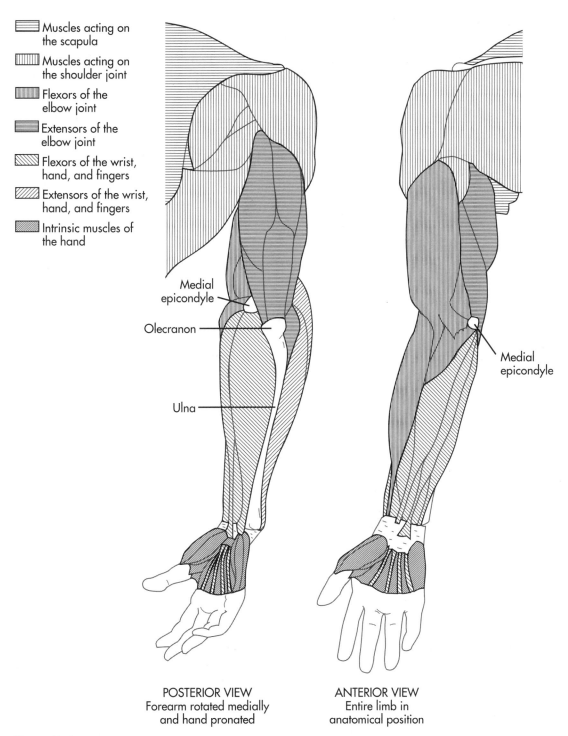

Muscles acting on the scapula

Muscles acting on the shoulder joint

Flexors of the elbow joint

Extensors of the elbow joint

Flexors of the wrist, hand, and fingers

Extensors of the wrist, hand, and fingers

Intrinsic muscles of the hand

Medial epicondyle

Olecranon

Ulna

Medial epicondyle

POSTERIOR VIEW
Forearm rotated medially
and hand pronated

ANTERIOR VIEW
Entire limb in
anatomical position

Figure **1.6**   Muscles of the upper extremity
(Note: Forearm muscles acting on the thumb are
not visible in this view.)

motion. Unfortunately, connective tissue has no way of differentiating between a desired posture and an undesired posture; it will organize itself along whatever line of tension the body imposes (Barnes, 1991). If an extremity is in a deformed posture secondary to abnormal muscle tone, muscle weakness, or skeletal malformations, the fascia will follow suit.

The types of fascia include superficial fascia, which connects the skin to the muscles; deep fascia, which is the visceral connective tissue; and dural fascia, which surrounds the brain and spinal cord. Fascia itself has both elastin fibers and collagen fibers. The elastin fibers promote elasticity and tissue memory, whereas the role of the collagen fibers primarily is for strength. These fibers are embedded in a gel-like substance, which plays a major role in fiber mobility. Fascia has the capacity to constrict and reconfigure itself around muscles and joints, which inhibits normal fluid movement.

Fascia has strong influences on the positioning and functioning of physically disabled children. In pediatric splinting, particularly when using serial splinting to gain range of motion at the various joints of the hand, the fascia should be assessed carefully for its role in the restriction or limitation of movement. We recommend that therapists with limited information on fascia refer to textbooks on myofascial release (see Appendix A).

## Arches

The bones of the hand are arranged into three arches. Two of the arches are transversely oriented, and one is longitudinal (Figure 1.7). The proximal transverse arch, which lies at the level of the distal carpals, is relatively fixed. The distal transverse arch, which lies at the metacarpal heads, is more mobile. During activity of the hand, this arch deepens (or curves) to assist with grasp and opposition of the thumb to the fingers. The longitudinal arch lies at the center of the hand and consists of the central carpal bones, the second and third metacarpals, and the index and middle fingers. The thumb, little, and ring finger rotate and move around the index and middle fingers, allowing the palm to cup or flatten to accommodate objects held in the hand.

To a large degree, the intrinsic muscles of the hand are responsible for maintaining the configuration of the arches. A collapse in the arch system may result from injury to the osseous skeleton, abnormal muscle tone, or paralysis or weakness of the intrinsic muscles. Arches are necessary for functional use of the hand.

In our experience with pediatric patients, we have noticed that the arches of the hand frequently can become flattened and immobile. Long-standing disabilities, which include limited functional use of the hand or severely increased or decreased muscle tone, can lead to changes in the arches and severe functional problems in the hand. When selecting splints in pediatric or developmental settings, remember that many of these patients have never experienced typical development and use of the hand and its arches. This factor can be significant when deciding the types of splints to be fabricated throughout the child's years of therapeutic intervention. Splints that support the arches not only provide improved anatomical alignment, but enable the child to have better hand function.

The arches of the hand in combination with the metacarpal bones of the fingers, which are different lengths, result in the formation of two oblique angles when an object is grasped in the hand. This principle is known as dual obliquity and must be considered

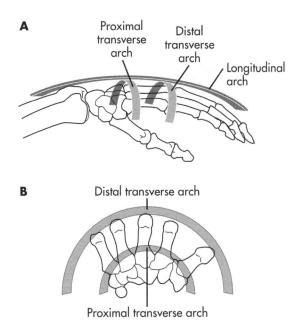

**A**

Proximal transverse arch

Distal transverse arch

Longitudinal arch

**B**

Distal transverse arch

Proximal transverse arch

Figure **1.7** The three skeletal arches of the hand. **A,** lateral view; **B,** transverse view

when fabricating splints that support any portion of the second through fifth metacarpal bones. From a dorsal perspective of the hand, dual obliquity results in an oblique angle from the metacarpal heads to the longitudinal axis of the forearm (Figure 1.8). From a transverse view, the metacarpal bones create an oblique angle in the transverse plane of the forearm. The object grasped in the hand is not parallel to the floor when the forearm is pronated (Figure 1.9). In addition, the radial side of the hand is higher than the ulnar side, and the fingers, when flexed, angle toward the radial side of the hand.

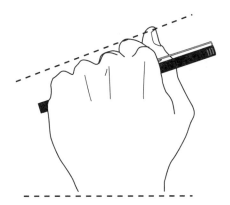

Figure **1.8** Dual obliquity, dorsal perspective

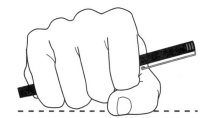

Figure **1.9** Dual obliquity, transverse view

Copyright © 1987. Fess, E. E., & Philips, C. A. *Hand splinting principles and methods.* St. Louis, MO: Mosby. Reprinted with permission.

## Anatomical Landmarks

Creases are wonderful landmarks for clinicians who fabricate splints. They provide helpful information regarding functional movement patterns of the hand. By either splinting over or clearing a crease, you can restrict undesired movement or allow desired movement. There are several important creases in the hand (Figure 1.10).

Starting distally, there are three sets of creases on the palmar surface of the phalanges: the distal digital creases (over the distal interphalangeal [IP] joints), the middle digital creases (over the proximal IP joints), and the proximal digital creases (slightly distal to metacarpophalangeal [MP] joints). The thumb has two creases: the metacarpophalangeal crease located over the MP joint and the interphalangeal crease located over the IP joint. The palm of the hand has four creases: the distal palmar transverse crease, the proximal palmar transverse crease, the middle palmar crease, and the thenar crease. The wrist has creases as well. While there are actually three, frequently they are grouped as one. On an infant, there often is only one visible crease due to the layer of "baby fat." On some infants and young children, this crease is continuous across the entire surface of the wrist for the same reason. The final significant crease of the upper extremity is the one at the elbow.

The thenar crease plays a significant role when fabricating splints for children. Many children who need splints have neuromuscular disabilities and frequently have spasticity in the adductors and flexors of the thumb. The movements of the thumb include flexion and extension (or radial abduction), abduction (or palmar abduction) and adduction, and rotation to oppose the four fingers.

Other important landmarks when splinting are the bony prominences in the upper extremity. The clinician should be aware of these to ensure that the splint is comfortable and will not cause any surface tissue injury. Knowledge of these potential problem areas is particularly important when splinting children or developmentally disabled adults who may not be able to tell you that they are in pain. Be aware of two primary bony prominences of the forearm, the ulnar styloid process and the styloid process of the radius. They can be seen on the dorsal surface and should be monitored closely when dorsal or circumferential wrist splints are used. This ensures that pressure sores do not develop. The pisiform bone (one of the carpal bones, palpated in the palm proximal to the little finger and just distal to the wrist crease), the lateral head of the MP of the index finger, the olecranon process (the elbow), and the lateral and medial epicondyles of the humerus are five more bony areas that are prone to pressure sores when they are splinted.

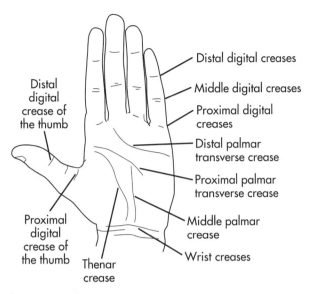

Figure **1.10**  Creases in the hand

## Development of the Hand

There are two aspects of normal development with which the pediatric therapist must be familiar not only to fabricate functional pediatric splints but, on a more elementary level, to establish effective treatment programs for children. First, the clinician must understand the progression of normal grasp and pinch patterns. This includes knowledge of different functional uses of the hand and arm, such as pointing, waving, and touching. Second, the therapist should be able to recognize and predict typical motor development of the non-disabled infant from birth through *at least* the first year. It is essential to know how gross-motor development affects the acquisition of fine-motor skills. A therapist who is well-grounded in normal development will not only be able to fabricate splints to meet the current needs of the patient, but also will be able to accurately assess the child's entire status and plan for the attainment of future developmental levels through therapy and splinting.

There are many notable textbooks on the development of prehension and grasp in infants and children (see Appendix A). Erhardt (1994) assesses voluntary grasp and pinch in terms relative to the type of objects that can be held: a dowel, a cube, a pellet, and a crayon or a pencil. Case-Smith (1995) defines hand-skill development during the first year in terms of "quartiles," or three-month periods during which the child integrates all the necessary components of development including posture, sensory processing, play, and cognitive development in order to master grasp, release, and bimanual skills.

Although clinicians may use different classification systems and terms to describe a particular type of pinch or grasp, there is general agreement on the major components of grasp development. First, there is clearly an order in which children acquire hand skills. Second, there are some necessary prerequisites to functional hand use, including adequate vision to see the object desired, enough control of the proximal portion of the extremity to enable the child to reach and place his hand near the desired object, the postural control to stay upright while reaching, adequate and appropriate sensation, and refined volitional control of the thumb, fingers, and wrist flexors and extensors.

Table 1.1 summarizes some frequently used terms in classification systems for prehension development in children up to age 15 months. (There are other types of grasp seen in toddlers and older children, including a variety of grasps used to hold writing utensils, a hook grasp, spheric grasp, cylindric grasp, and a lateral pinch.) If a type of pinch or grasp has more than one name, the table includes each name to help clarify differences between grasp-classification systems.

By age 1, a typically developing toddler has learned to grasp and release small objects, such as blocks or utensils, has learned to pick up a raisin with a fine-pincer grasp, can transfer objects from one hand to the other, and is beginning to scribble with a crayon or marker. However, children don't always acquire hand skills in a textbook manner. Frequently, a child "plays around" with new skill acquisition by practicing an emerging skill, reverting back to a more well-known and reliable skill when the mood strikes, and then practicing the new skill again until it becomes comfortable.

In addition to grasping and pinching, the hand has many other essential functions. Infants transfer objects from one hand to the other, bear weight on the upper extremities when crawling or sitting, and use their arms to pull themselves to standing. As infants get older they learn to release an object, then to throw, carry, and manipulate objects using two hands in a coordinated manner.

Table 1.2 summarizes some upper extremity and fine motor skills of infants and toddlers. They are performed in a predictable manner in the typically developing, non-disabled child. The development of these skills has direct application to your splint selection for a particular child. It is important, for example, not to select a forearm supination splint for a child less than 4 months of age because children don't typically use forearm supination with reach until that time. Refer to Appendix A for suggested readings on normal motor development.

The preschool child, like the adult, uses both power grasps and refined grasps. A power grasp involves extension at the wrist. The object is held in the palm and has significant contact with the palm and the volar surfaces of the fingers. The extrinsic muscles of the extremity are most active. There is strong thumb flexion and adduction. There is also strong flexion of the ring and small finger (Strickland, 1987). This type of grasp is used to push a manual wheelchair, pull up pants, brush hair, and pull a t-shirt down over the head. It usually is used in some variation to control the joystick on a power wheelchair. In a refined grasp, the position of the wrist is less important. The radial portion of the hand is most active, along with the intrinsic muscles. The object is out of the palm and is held skillfully through opposition between the thumb and the fingers (Strickland, 1987).

Table **1.1** **Classification of Prehension Development**

| Type of Grasp | | Typical Age Grasp is Seen | Description |
|---|---|---|---|
| **SQUEEZE GRASP** | | 4 to 5 months | The fingers flex the object against the palm. Motor control is crude, and the object is squeezed tightly. |
| **PALMAR GRASP** | | 5 to 6 months | The thumb is adducted, and the object is held actively with the fingers. |
| **INFERIOR-SCISSORS GRASP** | | 7 months | The child rakes the object with the fingers and attempts to grasp it by flexing all the fingers against a flexed thumb. |
| **RADIAL-PALMAR GRASP** | | 7 months | The thumb opposes the fingers and is used to hold the object. The object is in the palm. |
| **RADIAL-DIGITAL GRASP** | | 8 months | The thumb opposes the fingers, and the object is held in the hand outside the palm. The child first uses this grasp with a straight wrist and then an extended wrist. |
| **SCISSORS GRASP** | | 8 to 9 months | The thumb holds an object against the lateral side of a flexed index finger after a raking movement of the fingers. There is no opposition at the thumb. |
| **INFERIOR-PINCER GRASP** | | 9 months | The thumb is beginning to oppose an object and holds it between the distal pad of the thumb and the volar surface of the index finger. |
| **THREE-JAWED CHUCK GRASP** | | 10 months | The object is held outside the hand between the pads of the thumb, index, and middle fingers. |
| **PINCER GRASP** | | 10 months | The thumb opposes the index finger and holds the object between the distal pads of the thumb and index finger. |
| **TIP PINCH, FINE PINCER GRASP, OR SUPERIOR PINCER GRASP** | | 12 months | The most refined pinch, the child opposes the thumb and index finger as in the pincer grasp, but the object is held at the distal tips near the fingernails. The DIP of the thumb has significant flexion. |

Illustrations by Teresa Allison, OTR

Table **1.2** **Pediatric Upper Extremity Gross and Fine Motor Skills**

| Age Skill Appears | Upper Extremity Gross and Fine Motor Skill |
|---|---|
| Birth to 2 months | physiological flexion |
| 2 months | grasp reflex |
| 3 months | hands together on chest in supine position |
| 4 months | grasp reflex diminishing |
| | objects held in both hands at midline in supine position |
| | bears weight on forearms, more weight on the ulnar side than the radial side |
| | pats sides of bottle with hands |
| 5 months | two-handed approach to objects, but grasp is unilateral |
| | bilateral transfer |
| | extended-arm weight bearing in prone position |
| | places two hands on bottle with some forearm supination |
| 6 months | weight shifts on extended arms in prone position |
| | sits with a straight back |
| | elbows fully extend when reaching |
| 7 months | first purposeful release |
| | pulls self to stand |
| 8 months | crawls on hands and knees |
| 9 months | active forearm supination when reaching |
| 10 months | pokes with index finger |
| 12 months | uses hands in a coordinated manner in which one hand stabilizes and the other manipulates |
| | begins to scribble |
| 15 months | releases a pellet with wrist extension and precision |

Material in this table based on Bly, 1983; Erhardt, 1994; Case-Smith in Henderson and Pehoski, 1995; Case-Smith, Allen and Pratt, 1996; Morris and Klein, 1987.

This type of grasp is used to write, button clothing, finger feed, pick up a small object, or use utensils.

## Principles of Splinting and Fabrication

When it comes to splinting in pediatrics, clinicians have numerous design options. Although Chapter 4 provides you with information and patterns for as many types of splints as you're probably going to need, there will be occasions where you need to design your own splint or modify an existing pattern to meet the specific needs of your clients. It is likely you will find a pattern for an adult that you want to modify to fit a child's hand. Frequently, an adult pattern can be reduced on a photocopy machine until the desired size is obtained, needing only a few revisions.

However, after years of modifying adult patterns for children, we have discovered that the proportions of a child's wrist and hand aren't necessarily the same as those of an adult. An adult's forearm can be longer in proportion to the hand than a child's, and the forearm, hand, and fingers of a young child frequently are pudgy due to that layer of "baby fat." A basic understanding of the design principles of splinting will make it simpler to think on your feet and to make modifications for better fitting, more effective splints.

## Design and Fabrication

Analyzing splint design and fabrication principles from a scientific perspective can be confusing and overwhelming. Fortunately for most of us, there are a number of existing patterns available that will meet the needs of most of our patients. Yet, if a therapist is to fabricate an originally designed splint for a patient, it is essential to have an understanding of the elementary principles of splint design and fabrication. Once again, we refer you to the bibliography and Appendix A, this time for some suggested readings on hand-splinting principles. We recommend that you have at least one comprehensive splinting textbook on hand if you are custom designing a lot of splints. The information in this chapter summarizes some common principles.

In their most basic form, forearm splints can be classified as levers. The forearm trough provides a counter force to the distal portion of the splint over an axis point, which is the wrist. Splints are beneficial when there is an imbalance of internal forces in the hand or arm due to illness or injury. A splint can be defined as an external force used to correct imbalances. Both Hunt Kiel in *Basic Hand Splinting: A Pattern-Designing Approach* (1983) and Fess and Phillips in *Hand Splinting Principles and Methods* (1987) discuss numerous mechanical principles of splinting necessary for safe, effective, and comfortable splints. Several of their points are summarized below.

*Design the lever arm of the splint as long as possible to displace the pressure necessary to create the required force.* A splint must create force, but it must also be comfortable. The more surface area covered by a splint, the more comfortable it should be for a patient to wear. A splint that goes two-thirds of the way up the forearm and halfway up the sides of the forearm usually is adequate to displace the pressure and still be comfortable. Occasionally, when splinting a small child with "baby fat," the splint must be shorter than two-thirds of the way up the forearm to prevent the skin from being pinched when the elbow is flexed. (This caution also applies to obese patients.)

*The splint's points of pressure must be made as wide as possible on the patient's arm to disperse the pressure over the skin and decrease the chance of a pressure sore.* The more surface area the splint covers, the more evenly dispersed the pressure will be on the extremity, and the more comfortable the splint will be for the patient (Fess and Phillips, 1987). Splints made with a thermoplastic material with elastic or plastic qualities that conform to contours and creases in the hand disperse pressure evenly and can be quite comfortable for your patients to wear. (However, avoid pressure directly over bony prominences when possible to decrease the risk of pain and tissue damage.) In addition, wider straps disperse pressure better than do narrow straps.

*The axis point of pressure of the splint must always be exactly over the axis of the joint being splinted; all three points of pressure must be present and in the proper locations.* Typically, the splint and its straps work together to distribute the external forces of the splint onto the extremity. On a simple wrist cock-up splint, three straps usually are adequate: one proximal to the wrist on the forearm, one at the wrist, and one distal to the wrist. Frequently, when making small hand splints for infants and young children, the surface area is so small it is difficult to find enough room for three straps. In this situation, try cutting down a standard 1-inch piece of strap to 1/2 inch or 1/3 inch. You also can put a circumferential wrap around the entire splint to apply even pressure on the extremity. Don't eliminate a strap because there is not enough room for it if the strap is needed to apply pressure over the axis of the splint.

*If an unsplinted joint is to be allowed motion, the splint must not extend into the defined boundaries of the joint (including the skin creases).* Make sure that the proximal and distal ends of the splint are not so long as to interfere with your patient's available motion. If MP flexion is to be permitted, the distal palmar portion of the splint must clear the MP heads and the distal palmar transverse crease. It is a good practice not to "over splint" your patients. This means that if your patient, for example, has adequate thumb use but needs positioning and support at the wrist, select a splint that clears the thenar eminence and the MP and IP joints of the thumb so the thumb is free to move unrestricted.

*The splint should allow for normal anatomical properties.* These include placement in a functional position, support of the arches of the hand, allowance for dual obliquity, and allowance for all possible prehension patterns given the design of the splint being used. You must keep in mind the anatomy of the upper extremity when splinting it and applying straps so you don't apply inappropriate force on any ligaments, accidently flatten the arches, or force the bones into an unintended alignment.

*The importance of selecting the correct material for your splint, based on its intended purpose, cannot be overstated.* Splinting materials have different qualities and characteristics. They are manufactured to respond to force and handling in different ways. The type of material selected will play a major role in the success or failure of the splint. For example, some splinting materials are designed to bend with the child if the child has a muscle spasm. If a very rigid material is selected for a splint of this nature, the child will experience a lot of discomfort during the spasm, and depending on the strength of the muscle spasm, the fingers might pull out from under the straps. If a less rigid material is used, the splint could break. In addition, materials come in varying thicknesses, which also affect the strength of the material. Aside from always opting to use a thick material to increase strength, you can add contour to your splints whenever possible in order to increase the material strength mechanically (Fess and Phillips, 1987). Perforated materials will allow some air to get to your patient's skin, but they can weaken the splint if you overstretch the perforations while you are fabricating. Refer to Chapter 2 for descriptions of various splinting and strapping materials.

## Splint Classification Systems

In addition to understanding splint design and fabrication, you need to understand the different types of splints you might make. Just as there are a number of grasp-classification systems, there are a number of splint-classification systems. We like the splint-classification system that Roholdt (1994) uses: static, serial static/static progressive, dynamic, drop out, and articulated. Her differentiation between static and serial static/static progressive is particularly helpful. Yet Roholdt does not specifically address the use of neoprene, which has become a standard splinting material within pediatric populations. Soft materials such as neoprene can add an element of mobility to an otherwise static design. Hill (1988) addresses the use of neoprene materials. She has only three types of splints in her classification system: dynamic, semidynamic, and static. In their book *Hand Splinting Principles and Methods* (1987), Fess and Phillips introduce a new method of splint classification based on force complexity, joints involved, and kinematic purpose.

We haven't found that the lack of a universally accepted splint classification system has affected the functional benefits of our splints, but it can make it difficult to communicate the type of splint being fabricated to other professionals. It seems that neoprene has thrown a wrench into some of the existing classification systems. Additional confusion results from the fact that some systems are based on what the splint does, some on the joints it involves, and some on what the splint is made of.

After examining the existing classification systems, we developed one we think works well for pediatrics. It combines existing definitions with the use of neoprene, and it incorporates categories for commonly used pediatric splints. It includes the three categories Hill identifies: dynamic, semidynamic, and static, and adds two subcategories to static from Roholdt: serial static and static progressive. Examples of these categories are found in Chapter 4.

### Dynamic splints

These splints achieve their effect by imposing movement and force. They have extrinsic moving parts. They are used to compensate for muscle function, correct contractures, protect surgical repairs, and provide exercise for weak muscles. Dynamic splints frequently are associated with adjustable force via springs or rubber bands, high- and low-profile outriggers, cuffs, and hooks. A "typical" dynamic splint rarely is used with children for several reasons. First, they contain small parts and protruding objects and are generally considered unsafe for children. Second, the rehabilitation treatment program that usually accompanies dynamic splinting requires a level of cognition and responsibility that young children may not have. A dynamic splint may be necessary if a child receives a nerve or tendon injury or has some type of tendon transfer, but these situations are uncommon in the pediatric rehabilitation setting. If a dynamic splint is required, therapists should do their best to eliminate small, detachable pieces and high-profile outriggers. Thera-Band® Tubing™ can be substituted for rubber bands to help reduce the risk of choking. The simpler the design, the better. The dynamic elbow flexion splint is one type of dynamic splint that we like. It is low-profile and has limited detachable parts.

### Semidynamic splints

While these splints have no externally applied moving parts, they do have mobilizing forces that act on the hand. They are fabricated in part or in whole from neoprene and other soft or elastic-like materials that give and pull. They position the hand for improved function and allow active movement of the extremity. They also can provide support to the hand during use and correct or prevent deformity. These splints commonly are used in a pediatric setting. Examples include the sof-splint and a range of neoprene thumb abduction splints.

### Static splints

These splints have no moving parts. They provide positioning to rest a joint, support of the hand during use, protection from injury, positioning for improved function, and prevention or correction of deformity. They are typically worn when needed (during functional activity) or, in the case of resting a joint or preventing further deformity, on a regularly scheduled basis. They usually are made of thermoplastic materials. These splints commonly are used in a pediatric setting. Examples include both dorsal and volar wrist cock-ups, thumb spicas, and resting hand splints.

*Serial static splints.* These static splints, whose function is to use a low-load, long-duration stretch to make biological changes in the tissues of the extremity, are made of thermoplastic materials and have no moving parts. They are remolded or refabricated when significant changes in the joints or tissues have been achieved. These splints are used frequently in pediatrics, usually to increase passive range of motion. Examples include the circumferential wrist positioning and circumferential elbow splints.

*Static progressive splints.* These splints also are static splints with no moving parts. They have a design component that can be adjusted to allow for changes in joint position as range of motion improves. Static progressive splints can be made of neoprene or other soft materials, or a combination of soft materials and thermoplastics. As with the serial static splint, the intent is to make changes in the extremity and modify the splint when needed. In this type of splint, the basic form is not refabricated. Instead straps, hinges, or other mobile forces are modified, removed, or adjusted once moderate change has occurred. Examples include the wrist cock-up splint with neoprene thumb loop and the thumb abduction supination splint.

## Splinting in Pediatrics

You have a 4-year-old boy with spastic hemiplegia on your caseload. What type of splint should you fabricate? Unfortunately, there are no published protocols that will tell you which splint to make for your pediatric patients based on their diagnosis. However, some splints are more straightforward than others. Some are for a singular or very specific problem. Splints to manage scar tissue after a traumatic injury or a burn or for rehabilitation and healing following a surgical procedure have been designed for a specific set of problems, and their application is specific. In cases like these, while the post-surgical intervention and treatment approach are modified due to the age and cognitive skills of the child, the type of splint needed can be taken directly from the literature pertaining to adults. Only a few modifications for size, fasteners, and safety are needed. This is not to say that these splints are any easier to fabricate or require less skill, but splints for children with these needs can be located in existing texts on splinting. As in the case of burns and surgeries, there *are* protocols the therapist should obtain prior to splint fabrication. But splints for singular problems are probably the least common types of splints needed in the pediatric rehabilitation setting.

It is children with spasticity, muscle weakness, and joint problems who have diverse splinting issues for which it is a challenge and no protocols exist. It is these children for whom this book is written. It is important to analyze their total upper-extremity status and function completely before applying a splint.

## Making the Correct Splint Selection

The splinting needs of the children on the pediatric therapist's caseload can be singular, such as a splint that positions the wrist in extension yet frees the fingers to provide maximum independence while operating a joystick-control on a power wheelchair; or the needs can be multiple, such as a splint that opens a hand to provide adequate room for cleansing, stretches spastic wrist and thumb flexors, and allows soft tissues damaged from lack of adequate ventilation and cleansing to heal.

Where do you start when you receive a referral on a child with multiple needs? The key to selecting a proper splint in pediatrics is prioritizing. Unfortunately, it cannot be assumed that remediation of hygiene problems always precedes positioning problems or vice versa. Each child's problems necessitate personalized evaluation prior to the fabrication of the splint. There are situations in which a splint can be fabricated that meets all your patient's needs, but this usually isn't the case. The opposite is almost always true. A splint that tries to address all the needs of a complicated pediatric hand seldom meets any of the needs adequately. The best approach is to prioritize the needs, fabricate a splint that can correct the one or two most significant problems, and then periodically reassess the patient to see if a different splint should be fabricated to address what is now the most significant problem.

The importance of prioritizing the problems of each patient cannot be overemphasized. Some of the most common errors encountered by therapists with limited experience in pediatric splinting stem from the fantasy that they can fabricate a splint that will simultaneously meet all the needs of their patient. It is more beneficial for the patient to receive a splint that improves *some* of the problems in the hand than it is to have a splint that tries to improve *all* the problems at one time and therefore improves none. As children change and develop, their splinting needs and the types of splints used also will change. Sometimes the current splint can be modified, such as the addition of an elastomer insert to a neoprene thumb abduction splint. Sometimes children need to switch to a different splint as they develop, perhaps beginning with a circumferential wrist positioning splint and eventually changing to a dorsal cock-up splint. (These splints and modifications are all discussed in the subsequent chapters.) A splinting program is an ongoing process. A splint is not like a bath chair that can be recommended and expected to last the child for the next three years. Splints that do not fit properly or do not work appropriately can do more harm than good. They should be regularly monitored and modified or changed based on the individual needs of the patient.

## Using the Splint Selection Flow Chart

Although the problems with a particular child's hand can be numerous and diverse, our experience with children with physical disabilities has led us to conclude that there are four main reasons to fabricate a splint for a child's upper extremity. They are 1) to improve the positioning, 2) to improve the functioning, 3) to enable adequate hygiene, and 4) to protect the extremity or the child.

The Pediatric Splint Selection Flow Chart (Figure 1.11) demonstrates the system of prioritization and evaluation a therapist uses to determine which splint is most appropriate for the needs of the patient. Experienced therapists learn to follow this model in their heads. It is a mechanism for determining and prioritizing factors of primary importance, establishing a splinting goal, selecting a splint, and assessing the effectiveness of that splint for your patient.

The splint selection process described in this model is used in conjunction with the Priority Rating Form (Figure 1.12) found on page 25. The first step is to examine a series of "primary factors" that will enable you to establish a goal for the splint. The factors to consider fall under each of the four primary purposes for splinting listed at the top of the chart: positioning, function, hygiene, and protection/behavior. To examine these areas, consider the patient, and ask yourself the guiding questions under each

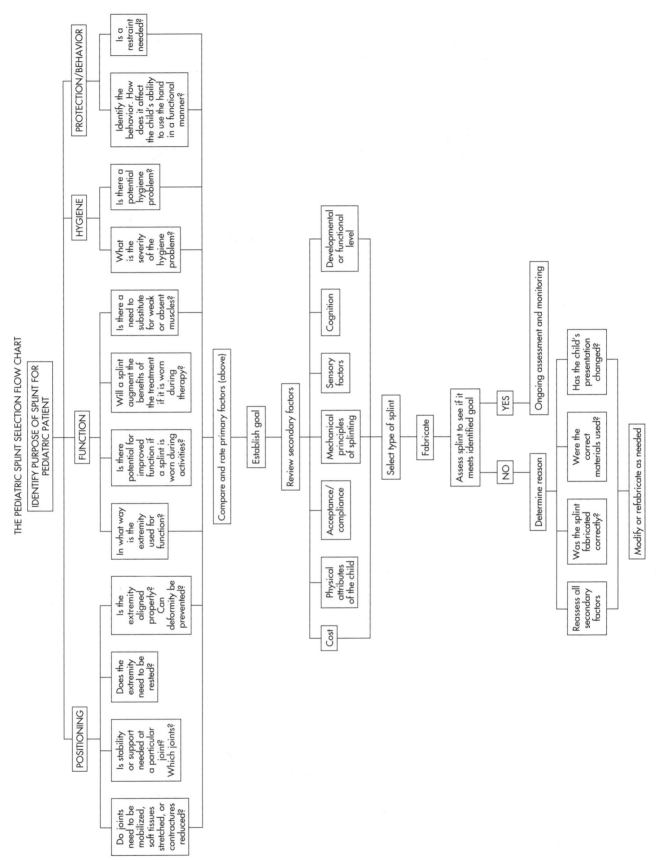

Figure **1.11** Pediatric Splint Selection Flow Chart

heading. The range of issues to be considered is broad: there may not be a concern in all the areas for every patient. If a particular area is not a concern, proceed across the flow chart and continue to address areas of importance for the individual patient. While going through the primary factors, record those that seem important on the Priority Rating Form.

Please note: Although the shoulder joint also is part of the upper extremity, it is not routinely splinted unless requested by the doctor following a surgical procedure, because of a burn, or in the case of a brachial plexus injury. The shoulder joint should always be assessed by itself for its role in function for the child such as weight bearing, reaching, or how it positions the distal extremity for function.

## Positioning

Under the category of positioning there are four points to be evaluated. The questions that follow address physiological changes that have occurred at the upper extremity. Problems related to positioning are often more obvious than other problems and can be the most difficult to splint.

1. *Do joints need to be mobilized, soft tissues stretched, or contractures reduced?* Look at each joint of the upper extremity: the elbow, wrist, thumb, and all the finger joints. First assess whether a contracture exists, and then determine the degree to which the contracture needs to be reduced. Try to determine what is causing the loss of range at each joint. Spasticity or shortened tendons can cause loss of range. The fascia surrounding the musculature of the extremity also can play a role in range problems. Constrictions in the fascia can be found at each of the joints. It is particularly common for the fascia of the palm to be constricted.

2. *Is stability or support needed at a particular joint? Which joints?* Assess each joint of the upper extremity to determine joint stability. Hypermobility of a joint decreases the stability and effectiveness of the joint for function. Hypermobility can be related to low tone and an accompanying lack of muscular stability at a joint. In other cases, however, such as in the hand of a child with spastic cerebral palsy, the MP and IP joints of the thumb become hypermobile due to excessive adduction and compensatory prehension patterns. Other joints of concern are the MPs of the fingers, which can become hypermobile as a compensatory means of opening the hand when wrist flexion is excessive. The wrist carpal bones can become hypermobile because of excessive flexion or ulnar deviation. While assessing stability and hypermobility of joints, you also should assess for dislocation or the potential for dislocation. Often a potential dislocation can be avoided through a splinting program that corrects the joint position before the joint becomes too compromised or damaged. If dislocation is suspected, you should refer the child to an orthopedist for an assessment or possible X-ray prior to fabrication of a splint.

3. *Does the extremity need to be rested?* Examine the upper extremity to determine if there is any swelling or pain. Determine if the upper extremity fatigues easily. When a joint is painful or swollen, active movement decreases and muscles can weaken. If movement decreases significantly, the joint can become stiff and immobile. Over time this leads to decreased active and passive range of motion and possibly more pain. Frequently the joints of children with juvenile rheumatoid arthritis are painful or sensitive to touch. These children often position their joints in a manner that decreases their pain but might impede function and lead to deformity.

4. *Is the extremity aligned properly? Can deformity be prevented?* Check the alignment of the joints of the upper extremity. See if the fingers are straight and if the wrist and forearm are in a neutral, functional position. Note the degree of available supination and pronation. Assess the joints during rest and then again during function to see if the child uses abnormal alignment to maximize functional use. Repetitive use of the hands and wrist in an abnormal position can lead to deformity. As you assess the child's upper extremity, keep in mind that the child is not fully grown. Children go through growth spurts that can affect the amount of force the muscles have over the joints. Poor alignment for a boy that has caused no significant problems over a period of years may become a concern when that boy enters puberty and gains muscle bulk and strength. This teenage boy may now be at risk for developing a deformity or contracture.

## Function

Under the category of function there are also four points to be evaluated. Upper extremity function is a critical area for the pediatric clinician to assess. It is important to have a clear understanding of the child's function prior to splinting to ensure that you don't accidently take away independent functioning by having the child wear a splint. If the needs for a splint to correct some other problem are more important than allowing the child to maintain some level of independent functioning, teach the child a new way to accomplish the task. If a child has a vital, functional skill he must perform and can no longer do with the splint on, it is likely he will discard the splint so he can continue his activity or wear it only occasionally. If the child is compliant and wears the splint, he could lose the ability to perform that functional activity.

1. *In what way is the extremity used for function?* Closely examine the child's current prehension patterns. Look at pinch and grasp, but also at other functional ways the child uses the extremity such as waving, pointing, or touching. Determine if new functional hand skills are emerging. Assess the potential to progress the child's current pinch or grasp to the next level. Determine if the extremity is functional despite alignment problems, or if corrective positioning at the thumb or wrist could improve function. For example, it is common to encounter excessive wrist flexion as a means for a child to obtain finger extension to grasp an object. Slightly more wrist extension would still allow the hand to open but would make the grasp stronger and more functional. It is also important to note whether you are assessing the child's dominant hand. If you are not and the child is independent with the dominant hand, you need to consider realistically how much you expect the child functionally to use the non-dominant hand. There is little sense in spending hours fabricating and coercing a young child into wearing a splint to align the pinch on his right hand, when his dominant left hand is totally functional. You may find, however, that an older child is more motivated to use the non-dominant hand and will willingly practice functional activities with the splint on.

2. *Is there potential for improved function if a splint is worn during activities?* Some children have learned to use their hands to accomplish all their necessary skills, with the exception of one or two tasks. It is amazing how much function a child can achieve through sheer motivation. Determine if the child would benefit from a splint with a singular purpose such as using the joystick on a power wheelchair, positioning the

wrist into some extension so that tenodesis will enable the child to maintain a tripod grasp on a pencil, or holding a non-adapted spoon at a restaurant. Try to determine which activities would allow the child to have increased independence if a splint were available. Sometimes the child or the family knows exactly what activity with which the child is having trouble. Be sure to ask them!

3. *Will a splint augment the benefits of the treatment if it is worn during therapy?* Determine if there are ways the child would benefit from a splint worn during therapy as part of the treatment process. Weight-bearing splints or positional thumb splints can be quite beneficial and will help you achieve other functional goals you have developed for the child. Typically, a splint fabricated for this purpose is not sent home and is worn only for brief periods of time during the day. Its purpose is to enable the child to practice and experience a movement, such as a pinch in the correct alignment or bearing weight on an open palm with proper arch support.

4. *Is there a need to substitute for weak or absent muscles?* Assess the functional muscle strength of the extremity. Identify which movements are unavailable to the child due to weakness. Usually, based on the diagnosis, you should be able to predict if weak muscles have the potential to interfere with function, and if so, if they will be in proximal or distal muscle groups. In addition to knowing whether the child has the strength to move his or her own body part, you should determine how much weight or resistance the extremity can handle or lift. This is important when selecting a functional splint because some splints are heavier than others.

## Hygiene

Under the category of hygiene there are two main areas to explore. When assessing hygiene, you are looking at the physical condition of the tissues of the extremity as well as the cleanliness of the extremity.

1. *What is the severity of the hygiene problem?* Examine the extremity to determine if there are any hygiene problems. Although there can be problems in the elbow crease and armpits, most frequently problems exist in the palm of the hand. Usually hands that are tightly fisted throughout the day are the ones that develop hygiene problems. One of the first things to look at when determining the severity of a hygiene problem is the color of the skin. Red skin indicates irritation. The skin may also appear blue or purple, indicating problems with circulation to the hand. Determine if there are signs of skin breakdown such as peeling or flaking skin, shiny and unhealthy-looking skin, or red marks or cuts from the fingernails. The child may be in pain as you attempt to open the hand to examine it. There may be bleeding or scabs caused by soft-tissue tears. Finally, tissues may have a bad odor caused by sweat or the inability of the caregiver to adequately clean the hand.

2. *Is there a potential hygiene problem?* Fortunately signs often are present in the child's hand to indicate that he or she is at risk for developing a hygiene problem. Look for moisture on the skin. The hand may be relatively clean but have dirt or dead skin between the fingers or in the palmar creases. This usually indicates the caregiver is having a difficult time cleaning the hand. Another candidate for a bad hygiene problem is the child with severely increased muscle tone or substantial contractures or the older child going through a growth spurt. These children's hands usually

are tightly fisted. If a hygiene problem is not already present, they are at risk for developing problems with the skin in the palm, particularly if the hand is sweaty and air does not circulate much through the palm.

## Protection/Behavior

In this category you are assessing factors related to the safety of the child. Identify behaviors the child demonstrates that may cause injury or directly interfere with functional hand use. Clinicians should become familiar with their facility's guidelines regarding splinting for protection of the child or behavioral concerns of the child. Sometimes a splint fabricated for a reason related to a child's behavior can be considered a restraint. Other times a splint fabricated to protect the hand of a child who, for example, bites herself, could lead to mouth injuries if she continues the same behavior but is now biting down on a hard splint. Deciding whether to make a splint for a child may boil down to an ethical decision on the part of the therapist. Assessing the following areas will help make the choice easier.

1. *Identify the behavior. How does it affect the child's ability to use the hand in a functional manner?* First, identify the behavior and the purpose it serves for the child. Although there are some behaviors demonstrated as a result of habit, most serve some purpose for the child. The child's behavior could be a result of a need to comfort himself, to receive sensory input, to release frustration, or a variety of other reasons. Find out how often the behavior occurs. It is possible the child is quite functional but you, the teacher, or the parent, grow tired of watching the behavior over and over and over again. Splints should not be fabricated to inhibit annoying behaviors that do not harm the child, but instead for functional reasons. For example, if you determine that a child mouths her hand for sensory input, and that when elbow flexion is blocked to prevent a hand-to-mouth action, she tolerates and participates in more socially acceptable sensory input such as touching soft materials or toys, then an elbow splint has a functional purpose. However, if elbow flexion is blocked and the child does not tolerate touching other textures and instead begins head banging, an elbow splint is not functional and may even be detrimental to the child's health.

2. *Is a restraint needed?* Sometimes a splint is not necessary. There are occasions when a child engages in behaviors that are a serious risk to his personal safety such as biting himself or poking his eyes with his fingers. In a case like this, a restraint to protect the child from injury may be needed. Find out who is responsible for such a decision and what the legal issues are regarding restraints in your state, community, and facility.

Table 1.3 summarizes the benefits of splinting for a pediatric population.

After you have examined these guiding questions, your answers must be evaluated and compared with each other. As you analyze the primary factors on the Splint Selection Flow Chart, those of concern should be listed, without respect to degree of importance, on the Priority Rating Form (Figure 1.12). Order does not matter at this point in the process.

When using the Priority Rating Form, compare each problem (or concern) you identified as you went through the guiding questions of the Splint Selection Flow Chart with every other problem. This process results in the identification of the primary goal(s) of the splint.

---

Table **1.3**    **Potential Benefits and Goals of Pediatric Splinting**

---

**POSITIONING**

Mobilize joints, stretch soft tissues, reduce contractures

Provide stability or support at specific joints

Rest the extremity

Provide proper alignment, prevent deformity

**FUNCTION**

Enable existing function to continue

Improve existing function

Augment benefits of therapy

Substitute for weak or absent muscles

**HYGIENE**

Improve a hygiene problem

Prevent a potential hygiene problem

**PROTECTION/BEHAVIOR**

Prevent or reduce the occurrence of an undesired behavior that interferes with functional upper-extremity use

Keep the child from injuring self

---

We will go through this process step by step using the example in Figure 1.13. The child's diagnosis is spastic quadriplegia with moderate to severe spasticity throughout the extremities and mild mental retardation. She is 8 years old. She has outgrown her current bilateral resting hand splints, which she wore throughout the day. When the occupational therapist evaluated her left hand for a splint the following were found to be primary concerns: 30° wrist-extension contracture; tight soft tissues in the palm; MP flexion contractures, 5° to 10° each on fingers 2 through 4; shiny, unhealthy skin in the palm; and reach but no grasp. In this example, the first step taken was to list the five

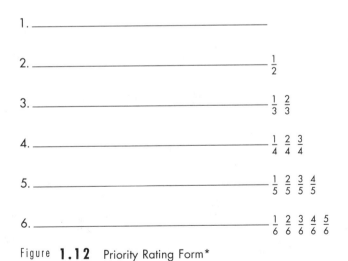

Figure **1.12**    Priority Rating Form*

---

*Copyright © 1994. *How to Manage Projects, Priorities and Deadlines Seminar.* National Seminars Group, a division of Rockhurst College Continuing Education Center. Reprinted with permission.

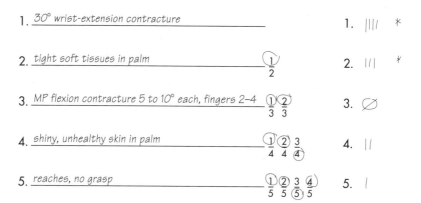

Figure **1.13**   Priority Rating Form for 8-year-old with spastic quadriplegia

problems in no particular order on the Priority Rating Form. They were numbered 1 through 5. You may identify any number of problems based on the specific needs of your patient.

The second step is to compare each problem to every other problem. Refer again to the sample in Figure 1.13. To begin, compare problem 1, 30° wrist-extension contracture, to problem 2, tight soft tissues in the palm. After comparing these two problems, the 30° wrist-extension contracture was determined to be more significant at this time. To record this, the 1 over the 2 was circled on the right side of the form. To continue, problem 1 was compared to problem 3, MP flexion contractures, 5° to 10° each on fingers 2 through 4. Of these two problems, 1 again was determined to be most significant. This was recorded by circling the 1 over the 3 on the right side of the form. Then, compare problem 2 to problem 3. Of these two problems, 2 was determined to be more significant. This was recorded by circling the 2 over the 3 on the right side of the page. Continue comparisons as shown in the sample until each problem has been compared to every other problem. Number 1 is compared to 4, 2 is compared to 4, and 3 is compared to 4. Number 1 is compared to 5, 2 is compared to 5, 3 is compared to 5, and 4 is compared to 5. If you have more than five factors, you would continue comparing them to each other and recording your opinions on the right side of the page.

By counting the total number of times each factor was circled on the right side of the form, you can determine the most important factor(s) to be considered when selecting a splint for your patient. In this example, the therapist determined the wrist-extension contracture to be the major concern for this patient, with tight palmar tissue being the second highest concern. Problem 1 was circled four times and problem 2 was circled three times. As a result of this process, the therapist established the splinting goal to be reducing wrist-extension contracture and increasing palmar mobility to prevent breakdown or injury to the palm. Whether the therapist plans to add this goal to the Individualized Educational Plan (IEP) or other treatment plan for the child is irrelevant. The actual goal related to the need for a splint may be to increase independence with power mobility. In most cases the goal will be a functional goal, and the splint will be considered part of the treatment plan to meet that goal. Regardless, as the clinician, you should have an idea of what you want the splint to accomplish in the next few months. In this example the therapist was able to prioritize the problems in the upper extremity of the patient and establish a goal for the splint. The other problems will be addressed by the splint only if they do not interfere with the ability to meet the established goal.

## Secondary Factors

Refer again to the Splint Selection Flow Chart (Figure 1.11). After identifying the goal of the splint, you must consider a set of "secondary factors," including types of material and design, that will assist further in the selection of the most appropriate splint. The secondary factors are not prioritized or compared to each other, but instead are used together to narrow the types of splints that could be used successfully for a particular patient. It is helpful to have an idea of the splint in mind when looking at these secondary factors. The secondary factors are as follows:

1. *Cost.* As expected, cost has a great deal of bearing on the type of splint selected for a patient. You need to know who is paying for the splint and what the payor's limits are. You may be able to purchase special materials for fabrication of the splint, or you may have to limit yourself to the ones in stock. Determine how frequently you anticipate the need to change or modify the splint. Other costs may need to be added. Also, the cost (or availability) of your time may need to be considered.

2. *Physical attributes of the child.* While tone and contractures already have been addressed to help identify the main goal of the splint, they will be addressed again here to help select the most appropriate splint or splinting material. Look at how much range is available to the child both actively and passively. It may be difficult to get the child positioned correctly into your splint of first choice because of muscle tone or range limitations. Significant limitations in finger extension may make a typical resting-hand splint difficult to get on the child. An IP contracture at the thumb may make it difficult to don a rigid thumb spica splint designed to immobilize the MP joint of the thumb. Assess the degree of abnormal muscle tone in the different muscle groups of the extremity. Find out if the child has frequent or severe muscle spasms. If so, you can fabricate a splint that can withstand the force of the muscle tone and spasms. Perhaps a thicker thermoplastic material or thicker neoprene is indicated. You also can select a material that bends with the child. Maybe a thinner or perforated elastic material with contour for strength will provide enough support but also bend with the child during a spasm. The presence of abnormal muscle tone significantly influences the type of material used.

   Assess the extremity to determine if all the anatomical structures are present. For example, if digits are missing, a standard pattern may have to be modified, and alternative strapping may have to be designed. Look for swelling and determine if it is a temporary or chronic condition. If it is temporary or occasional, you may have to apply padding to the splint to accommodate for changes in the size of the hand when the swelling has diminished.

   Other physical attributes of the child's upper extremity will help you determine if you need to fabricate a dorsal or volar splint. There are three main advantages to a dorsal splint. First, there is a better mechanical advantage if you are splinting the wrist. Second, the splint is less likely to move or shift on the hand. Third, there is less sweating on the dorsal surface of the hand. The main disadvantage of a dorsal splint stems from the fact that the dorsal surface of the forearm is bonier, and therefore there is a greater risk of pressure sores and injury to the soft tissues. There are also three main advantages to volar splinting. First, it is easier to block wrist flexion from the volar surface. Second, volar splints usually are easier to fabricate and often are preferred by therapists with less experience. Third, the volar surface has more natural padding, and there is a lower risk of pressure sores. The main disadvantage of volar splints is that there is often less surface area for straps. There have been several studies to determine whether or not a dorsal or a volar splint is better at reducing hypertonus. According to McPherson, Kreinever, Aalders, and Gallagher (1982), both types of static splints reduce hypertonus. Refer to Appendix 3 for more on this topic.

3. *Acceptance/compliance.* Therapists who have experience with splinting children already know that acceptance and compliance are major factors influencing the success of a splinting program. We have never met an adult patient who has thrown his splint out the window of a moving vehicle but we know many children who have! As the therapist, it is important that you find out if the child wants the splint. Find out if the child's peers or siblings are expected to be critical or approving of the splint. Peer recognition and approval influence children at a young age. If there are concerns that the child may be embarrassed to wear the splint, try to select and fabricate a splint that is more socially acceptable. Determine also if the parents or teachers want the splint. It is critical that the person responsible for donning the splint is compliant and able to follow directions. The last thing to find out is if the child has a history of removing splints at inappropriate times. If so, select a splint design that is difficult for a child to remove or choose strapping mechanisms that are not easily unfastened. Chapter 3 provides numerous tips and suggestions for making splints that are more socially acceptable as well as splints that are difficult for a child to remove.

4. *Mechanical principals of splinting.* Part of making the final selection for the splint is selecting the materials from which it will be made. Your selection can either enhance the splint or cause it not to work properly. After considering the physical attributes of the child, you must select the appropriate material for the splint, modify any aspect of the splint that may need customizing, and select the straps or fasteners. Based on the intent of the splint and how it will be worn, there are usually a few material choices available. If using an existing splint design, you may have to make modifications, such as deciding where to anchor straps on a tiny splint with little surface area, or customizing a finger pan for a child with individual, unique finger contractures. If the child has significant contractures and interference from muscle tone, you may have to notably modify a pattern if the splint is to be worn at all. If this is the case, be sure to incorporate the necessary design and fabrication principles (see previous section on mechanical principles of splinting).

5. *Sensory factors.* In a pediatric rehabilitation setting, children often are unable to verbally communicate about their well-being. This may be because they are too young to speak, or because they have a physical or cognitive impairment that impedes speech. A therapist needs to determine if the child is aware of personal comfort or experiences pain or discomfort when placed in the desired splinting position. This may influence the design of the splint or the material and strapping you select. Consider when the splint will be worn. If it is during a time when the child is in quadruped or otherwise needs to receive sensory feedback from the hands or forearms, you may want to select a dorsal splint or a neoprene splint.

6. *Cognition.* Another factor to be considered is cognition. If the child you are splinting has a low cognitive level, take extra caution by eliminating small pieces and avoiding

some glues or adhesives. Provide thorough information to the caregiver on fit and comfort. If the child's cognitive level is higher, you may be fabricating a splint that the child will don and doff independently. The child's cognitive level needs to be paired with the selection or design of the splint so that the child will be able to apply it correctly. The application of some splints, like a wrist cock-up with thumb hole, for example, is rather self-explanatory. In comparison, a serpentine splint looks different. People frequently confuse the dorsal and volar surfaces. Whenever possible the child should be told the purpose of the splint. This will increase compliance and help alleviate any fears the child may have about the splint.

7. *Developmental or functional level.* The therapist needs to consider the child's developmental level when deciding upon a splint. Consider the child's main environments. Perhaps the child is on the floor rolling or crawling around. Maybe the child is in a wheelchair the majority of the day with arms placed on a tray. The child may be ambulatory, playing with other children on the playground, taking care of most needs independently. These things need to be considered because the child's lifestyle will affect the type of splint you select. We have worked with children with hemiplegia, for example, for whom a resting-hand splint was probably an appropriate choice. Yet because these children were donning and doffing their own jackets and sweaters, the wide pan of the splint would have rendered them less independent as it is difficult to push it through the cuffs of sleeves. For these children, a close-fitting circumferential splint was selected. A weight-bearing splint may be the preferred splint for a young, preambulatory child, but its design may eliminate spontaneous transitions from crawling to fine-motor play. Because of this, a therapist may opt for a contoured thermoplastic thumb splint such as the thumb spica. This splint will not control the whole hand while bearing weight, but it will provide some proximal support and enable spontaneous fine-motor play.

These factors are summarized in Table 1.4.

After a little practice, you can review these primary and secondary factors in your head. Using this system will make splint selection easier. The following is an example of a splint selected for a 9-year-old boy with cerebral palsy and moderate spastic quadriplegia. Bill is right-hand dominant and has more spasticity on the left side than the right. After reviewing the 12 primary factors, you have determined that a left thumb splint is necessary to give him a more effective pinch and grasp on the left, which he uses spontaneously as an assist. While reviewing the secondary factors, you realize that compliance and social acceptance are significant factors influencing the success of previous splinting programs. (In other words, Bill takes off the splint and loses it about twice a month.) You may opt to fabricate a modified thumb-abduction splint out of a bright color of neoprene because it would resemble a bike glove, which the child thinks is "cool." But the standard thickness of neoprene may not control the thumb because it is held so tightly in the palm. You may then opt to purchase a thicker neoprene and use an elastomer insert at the web space. These material choices will solve your spasticity problem, but unfortunately, after further investigation of the secondary factors, you learn from your administrator that you have a $50 splinting budget for the entire year and $40 has been spent already. The splint you select for Bill, based on all the secondary factors, is a thumb spica out of an elastic material already stocked in your clinic. For $7 you purchase a set of permanent splint markers and have the child color the splint. He

Table **1.4** **Considerations Prior to Final Splint Selection**

**COST**
Limits of the payor
Amount of money allocated for the splint
Cost of the therapist's time

**PHYSICAL ATTRIBUTES OF THE CHILD**
Available range
Degree of muscle tone
Amount and severity of spasms
Anatomical structures present and intact
Swelling

**ACCEPTANCE/COMPLIANCE**
Person responsible for donning the splint is capable and compliant
Child and/or caregivers want the splint
Child will not remove the splint inappropriately

**MECHANICAL PRINCIPLES OF SPLINTING**
Correct materials are available
Splint is of sound design and applies appropriate forces and support

**SENSORY FACTORS**
Child's comfort taken into consideration
Splint does not interfere with necessary sensory feedback

**COGNITION**
Child will be safe while wearing the splint
Child understands purpose of the splint
Child can don the splint independently if needed

**DEVELOPMENTAL OR FUNCTIONAL LEVEL**
Splint will not interfere with child's current functional level

and his best friend write on the straps with fabric paint you found in the craft bins at the clinic. For added security you add an anti-Houdini fastener such as a safety webbing buckle (see Chapter 3 for more fastener ideas).

After the goal has been established and the secondary factors have been considered, you can turn to the Problem-Based Splint Selection Chart (Table 1.5) for help in selecting an appropriate splint and suggestions for recommended materials. The chart contains numerous possibilities for splint fabrication. You can easily identify the splint of choice, or if two or more will work equally well, pick the splint of preference (we all have our personal favorites and there is nothing wrong with using them if they meet the child's needs). Using this chart, you will make splint selections from a problem-based rather than diagnosis-based approach. Because no two children with the same diagnosis present with the exact same clinical picture, it is critical that you splint the problem and not the diagnosis.

This chart obviously is not all-inclusive. It is intended to assist the novice splinter but may also be helpful to those with more advanced skills. It lists commonly seen clinical problems (i.e., wrist flexion, thumb in palm, and limited forearm supination) and suggests a type of splint that has been found to be successful in correcting that problem.

Table **1.5** **Problem-Based Splint Selection Chart**

| Problem | Suggested Splint(s) | Suggested Material(s)** |
|---|---|---|
| **LIMITED ACTIVE ELBOW FLEXION** | a. Dynamic Elbow Flexion | a. Orthoplast (N,S) for harness, any thermoplastic for hand splint, latex tubing |
| **ELBOW FLEXION DEFORMITY** | a. Volar Elbow Extension<br>b. Circumferential Elbow<br>c. Soft Elbow Extension | a. Any rigid thermoplastic<br>b. Orfit, soft, 1/12" (N)<br>c. Polyurethane foam, orthopedic felt, etc. |
| **LIMITED FOREARM SUPINATION** | a. Forearm Serpentine<br>b. Forearm Serpentine with Neoprene Strap<br>c. TAP(R)/TASS | a. Aquaplast (R)<br>b. Aquaplast (R) and neoprene<br>c. Neoprene |
| **LIMITED FOREARM PRONATION** | a. Reverse TAP (R)/TASS | a. Neoprene |
| **WRIST RADIAL DEVIATION** | a. Long Thumb Spica<br>b. Volar Wrist Cock-Up with Radial Bar<br>c. Dorsal Wrist Cock-Up | a. Aquaplast (R)<br>b. Any thermoplastic<br>c. Aquaplast (R) |
| **WRIST ULNAR DEVIATION** | a. Neoprene Thumb-Abduction with Ulnar Gutter Insert<br>b. Volar Wrist Cock-Up with Thumb Hole<br>c. Dorsal Wrist Cock-Up | a. Neoprene with elastic or plastic insert<br>b. Any thermoplastic<br>c. Aquaplast (R) |
| **WRIST FLEXION** | a. Volar Wrist Cock-Up<br>b. Volar Wrist Cock-Up with Radial Bar<br>c. Dorsal Wrist Cock-Up<br>d. Circumferential Wrist Positioning<br>e. Volar Wrist Cock-Up with Thumb Hole<br>f. Resting-Hand | a. Any thermoplastic<br>b. Any thermoplastic<br>c. Aquaplast (R)<br>d. Orfit, soft, 1/12" (N)<br>e. Any thermoplastic<br>f. Plastic or plastic-rubber thermoplastic |
| **FISTED HAND** | a. Circumferential Wrist Positioning<br>b. Volar Anti-Spasticity<br>c. Dorsal Anti-Spasticity<br>d. Resting-Hand (with or without finger separators)<br>e. Palm-Protector Cone Splint<br>f. Palmar Hygiene<br>g. MacKinnon's | a. Orfit, soft, 1/12" (N)<br>b. Plastic or plastic-rubber thermoplastic<br>c. Plastic or plastic-rubber thermoplastic<br>d. Plastic or plastic-rubber thermoplastic<br>e. Plastic or rubber thermoplastic<br>f. Perforated elastic thermoplastic<br>g. Elastic or plastic thermoplastic, vinyl tubing |
| **THUMB IN PALM** | a. Sof-splint<br>b. Standard Neoprene Thumb-Abduction Splint<br>c. Thumb Spica<br>d. Hand-Based Serpentine<br>e. Saddle Splint<br><br>f. Modified Palmar Hygiene<br>g. Volar Wrist Cock-Up with Thumb-Abduction Loop<br>h. Long Thumb Spica | a. Neoprene<br>b. Neoprene<br>c. Elastic thermoplastic<br>d. Aquaplast (R)<br>e. Any thermoplastic, elastomer (N,R,S), Adapt-It pellets (R), X-Lite/Hexcelite (N,R)<br>f. Perforated elastic<br>g. Any thermoplastic and neoprene<br>h. Aquaplast (R) |
| **DOES NOT BEAR WEIGHT THROUGH AN OPEN HAND** | a. Clamshell (with pellet or putty mold base)<br>b. Mitt Weight-Bearing<br>c. Palmar Arch Orthosis<br>d. Inhibitive Weight-Bearing Mitt (IWM) | a. Aquaplast, solid and perforated (R), Adapt-It pellets (R)<br>b. Elastic, plastic or plastic-rubber thermoplastic<br>c. Any thermoplastic, Adapt-It pellets (R), elastomer (N,R,S) or neoprene<br>d. Plywood, plaster, Velfoam (N,R,S) or neoprene |

**N = North Coast Medical; R = Rehabilitation Division, Smith & Nephew, Inc.; S = Sammons Preston
Those materials listed under the Suggested Materials column are only personal recommendations. A similar material from the same thermoplastic category (i.e., elastic, plastic, rubber, plastic-rubber) may work just as well. We encourage you to experiment with several materials from different product vendors to determine which materials are the most appropriate for your clients.
Copyright © 1998 by Therapy Skill Builders, a division of The Psychological Corporation. All rights reserved/Laura Hogan and Tracey Uditsky, Pediatric Splinting/ISBN 0761615148/1-800-228-0752/This page is reproducible.

Use the recommended splints as a starting point and as a working tool. As you become experienced with pediatric splinting, you will inevitably modify existing patterns and even create your own designs. Add to the chart and delete from it as your clinical experience provides you with splint design and material preferences. Patterns and fabrication instructions for these suggested splints can be found in Chapter 4 with the exception of two splints, the inhibitive weight-bearing mitt (IWM) and the MacKinnon's. If you are interested in fabricating either of these splints, detailed instructions can be found in the articles referenced at the end of this book (Lind, 1992, and MacKinnon, Sanderson, and Buchanan, 1975).

Once the splint has been fabricated, you are not quite finished. Remember, splinting is a *process*. After fabrication you must again assess it to ensure that the splint is meeting its identified goal. Refer a final time to the Splint Selection Flow Chart (Figure 1.11) on pg. 20. Depending on whether or not the splint meets its identified goal, you can follow the chart and 1) continue to provide ongoing monitoring or 2) identify the reason the splint is not meeting its goal and make modifications or refabricate as needed. Usually a lack of success can be narrowed to one of four reasons, none of them fatal or irreparable. First, the secondary factors may not have been assessed correctly. Possibly there were factors unknown until the final fabrication of the splint. Second, the splint may not have been fabricated correctly. (Don't despair, fabrication does get easier with time and practice.) Third, the correct materials may not have been used to fabricate the splint. Splints have design features that require the material selected to display characteristics such as rigidity, flexibility, etc. An incorrect material selection will result in a less effective splint. Fourth, the child's presentation may have changed. The primary factors may have lessened or worsened, or the correction of the most significant factor may have led the therapist to discover a more significant factor now interfering with the splint's success.

# Materials

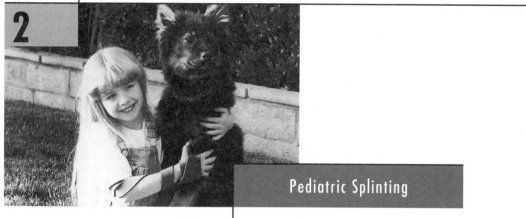

## Chapter 2

Pediatric Splinting

## History of Thermoplastics

Prior to the 1960s, hand splints were fabricated primarily from plaster of Paris, wood, steel, iron, or aluminum. Working with these materials was cumbersome and time-consuming, and the finished product was often heavy and bulky to wear. The introduction of high-temperature thermoplastics such as Royalite® and Plexiglas™ was a noted improvement. However, in order to soften these materials, a 500° oven was required, and the splints had to be fabricated using a positive-cast mold. Even after all this effort, the contour of the finished product still was poor, and edge finishing could be accomplished only through use of sandpaper and metal files.

In 1964, the first low-temperature thermoplastic, Prenyl®, was introduced. Prenyl was manufactured by Johnson & Johnson, and soon after its introduction, it had competition from other low-temperature thermoplastics such as Aquaplast®, Orthoplast® and Polyform®.

## Low-Temperature Thermoplastics

Today, the low-temperature thermoplastics on the market number about 35 and are ever-changing. For ease in understanding, we have broken the thermoplastic materials into four main types: 1) elastic-like, 2) plastic-like, 3) rubber-like, and 4) plastic-rubber-like. It is important to understand the qualities inherent in each type of material rather than memorize the characteristics of each brand name. In general, the characteristics and working properties of each type of thermoplastic will be similar, and if you have a general understanding of elastic-like materials, for example, you will be somewhat familiar with the working properties of each brand name that falls into the elastic-like category. Obviously it is less time-consuming to learn four categories than 35 brand names.

There is no one splinting material appropriate for all splinting needs. To be successful at splinting you must understand the characteristics or qualities that define materials as well as the working properties of each of the types of materials. Following is a brief description of the four main characteristics that define thermoplastic materials. These characteristics include: 1) drapability/conformability, 2) stretch and control, 3) memory, and 4) rigidity.

## Characteristic Definitions

The following characteristic definitions generally are accepted as described by the product manufacturers.

### Drapability/conformability

These interchangeable terms refer to the ability of the thermoplastic material to conform to the body part being splinted. When a material drapes or conforms easily to anatomical contours and arches, it is considered to have a high level or degree of drapability/conformability. Select a highly conforming material for use with burn management, bony areas, facilitation or enhancement of palmar arches, and precise positioning.

### Stretch and control

These terms refer to the amount of resistance to being stretched the material gives when it is heated. When a material stretches easily, it is considered to have a high level or degree of stretch and therefore, an accompanying low degree of control. Select materials with a high degree of stretch for small intricate splints, and avoid them for larger splints or splints to be fabricated on a child with severe spasticity.

### Memory

This refers to the ability of the heated material to return to its original shape after being stretched. It also refers to the inherent ability of the finished product to return to its original shape or pattern after it has been completely cooled and then reheated (serial splinting). When a material easily returns to its original shape, it is considered to have a high level or degree of memory and may be referred to as having "good memory." Select a material with good memory when you anticipate that frequent remolding and repositioning will be necessary.

### Rigidity

This refers to the strength of the thermoplastic material in its finished, cooled form. When a material maintains its original shape and resists bending and cracking, it is considered to have a high level or degree of strength or rigidity. Select a highly rigid material for children with spasticity or prolonged contractures.

Now, with an understanding of the characteristics that define thermoplastics, we will give an overview of the inherent working properties of each of the four types of thermoplastic materials: 1) elastic-like, 2) plastic-like, 3) rubber-like, and 4) plastic-rubber-like.

## Types of Materials

### Elastic-like

This group of materials has excellent memory. They have a high degree of conformability and a moderate-to-high degree of control or stretch. Elastics tend to resist fingerprinting, and the finished product is moderately rigid. Because of their excellent memory, elastics are a cost-effective and time-efficient choice for serial static splinting. The same splint can be reheated and remolded a number of times as soft tissue changes or improvements in range of motion or alignment are made. A common clinical example of an elastic material is Orfit®, Aquaplast®, or Prism™.

### Plastic-like

This group of materials has a high degree of conformability/drapability and stretch. They have low memory, fingerprint easily, and are strong/rigid in their finished form. Because of its high level of conformability and stretch, this type of material can be a good choice for intricate finger and hand splints that require a lot of contouring. Plastics are difficult to control, and therefore are not a good choice for therapists with limited splinting experience, for splints that need to cover a large surface area, or for use with spastic or uncooperative children. A common clinical example of a plastic material is Clinic® or Polyform.

### Rubber-like

This group of materials has a high degree of control and resists stretch. Therefore it has little drapability/conformability. Rubber-like materials have moderate memory and highly resist fingerprinting. The degree of rigidity varies among individual brands. These materials are a good choice for large splints that do not require a close fit. They also are a good choice for patients with spasticity because they have a high degree of control, and you can work aggressively with them without fingerprinting. A common clinical example of a rubber material is Synergy®, Orthoplast®, or Ezeform®.

### Plastic-rubber-like

This group of materials is known as being "middle of the road." They have a moderate degree of control and conformability, a moderate degree of memory, and moderate resistance to fingerprinting. Plastic-rubber materials are "user friendly" and are a good choice for therapists new to splinting or for clinics that cannot afford to stock materials in each of the four categories. A common clinical example of a plastic-rubber material is Preferred® or Polyflex II®.

Table 2.1 is intended as a quick reference guide to assist therapists with material selection. The majority of these thermoplastic materials can be purchased through North Coast™ Medical, Rehabilitation Division, Smith & Nephew Inc., and Sammons™ Preston; however, do not overlook some of the smaller, less-publicized companies. Although the variety of splinting materials is not as large at the smaller companies, the cost is often less for those products that they do carry.

In addition to sheets of thermoplastic materials, there are other low-temperature thermoplastic products that are useful in pediatric splinting. These include Aquaplast Ultra Thin™ Edging Material, Adapt-It Thermoplastic Pellets, and X-Lite® (Hexcelite®).

## Aquaplast Ultra Thin Edging Material

Aquaplast Ultra Thin Edging Material can be purchased in either sheets or strips. The 3/4-inch × 25-foot strip tends to work best for most pediatric purposes. The edging is made of a thin Aquaplast material. To use it you can pre-cut a piece in the desired length and heat it in water (160°–170°) or dry heat it with a heat gun until the strip becomes clear. Once the piece is clear, you quickly fold it over any splint edge that needs to be

Table **2.1** **Materials Reference Chart**

| Material Name** | Does It Conform/ Drape? | Does It Resist Stretch? | Does It Have Memory? | Does It Resist Fingerprints? | Is the Finished Product Rigid? |
|---|---|---|---|---|---|
| **ELASTIC-LIKE** | | | | | |
| Orfit, soft (N) | Yes | Some | Yes | No | No |
| Orfit, stiff (N) | No | Some/Yes | Yes | No/Some | No |
| Aquaplast Original (R) | Yes | Some | Yes | Yes | Semi |
| Aquaplast-T and Watercolors (R) | Some | Some | Yes | Yes | Semi |
| Aquaplast ProDrape-T (R) | Yes | No | Yes | Yes | Semi |
| Aquaplast Original Resilient (R) | Some | Some | Yes | Yes | Semi |
| Aquaplast Resilient-T (R) | Some | Some | Yes | Yes | Semi |
| Encore (N) | Yes | Yes | Yes | Yes | Semi |
| Kay-Plast (S) | Yes | Some | Yes | Yes | Semi |
| Multiform Clear Elastic (A) | Some | Some | Yes | Yes | Semi |
| Prism (N) | Yes | Some | Yes | Yes | No |
| **PLASTIC-LIKE** | | | | | |
| Clinic (N) | Yes | Some | No | No | Yes |
| Clinic D (N) | Yes | Some | No | No | Yes |
| Kay Splint Basic I (S) | Yes | No | No | Some | Yes |
| Kay Splint Basic II (S) | Yes | Some | Some | Some | Semi/Yes |
| Multiform Plastic (A) | Yes | No | No | No | Yes |
| Polyform (R) | Yes | No | No | No | Yes |
| Orthoplast II (S) | Yes | Some | No | Some | Semi/Yes |
| **RUBBER-LIKE** | | | | | |
| Synergy (R) | No | Yes | Some | Yes | Semi/Yes |
| Omega Plus (N) | No | Yes | Some | Yes | Semi/Yes |
| Spectrum (N) | No | Some/Yes | Some | Yes | Semi |
| Orthoplast (S) | No | Yes | Some | Yes | Semi |
| Ezeform (R) | Some | Yes | Some | Yes | Semi/Yes |
| Kay-Prene (S) | No | Yes | Some | Yes | Yes |
| Kay Splint IV (S) | Some | Yes | Yes | Yes | Semi |
| San Splint (R) | No | Yes | Some | Yes | Yes |
| **PLASTIC-RUBBER-LIKE** | | | | | |
| Kay Splint Basic III (S) | Some | Some/Yes | Some | Some | Semi/Yes |
| Preferred (N) | Some | Some | Some | Some | Semi |
| Polyflex II (R) | Some | Some | Some | Some | Semi/Yes |

**N = North Coast Medical; R = Rehabilitation Division, Smith and Nephew, Inc.; S = Sammons Preston; A = AliMed, Inc.

smoothed. If the strip starts to go opaque while you are working with it, use the heat gun or hot water to reheat it. This edge-finisher creates a durable, smooth edge that is extremely comfortable to the touch. This technique is especially helpful when finishing the edges of a splint that was fabricated with a perforated material or a splint that was fabricated with X-Lite because these materials have inherently rough edges.

Copyright © 1998 by Therapy Skill Builders, a division of The Psychological Corporation. All rights reserved/Laura Hogan and Tracey Uditsky, Pediatric Splinting/ISBN 0761615148/1-800-228-0752/This page is reproducible.

## Adapt-It Thermoplastic Pellets

Traditionally, Adapt-It Thermoplastic Pellets are used for adapting household items, such as building up handles on utensils or grooming aids, or for extending joysticks and wheelchair brakes. The pellets are available in one-pound or three-pound bags, are easy to use, and have 100% memory. Soften the pellets in hot water just as you would a sheet of low-temperature thermoplastic material. When the pellets become clear, remove them with a spatula and knead them together to form a mass of pliable putty. At this point, you have about 4 minutes of working time to be creative. If you use your imagination, you will find that these pellets offer many possibilities. Some of the more common uses that are especially helpful with pediatric splinting follow.

### Finger separators

Using Adapt-It Thermoplastic Pellets to fabricate finger separators, a customized fit easily is achieved. One common use is to add finger separators to the pan of a resting-hand splint. After the hand splint is fabricated and completely hardened, finger separators can be made by adding a softened mass of pellets directly to the splint pan portion. Next, place the patient's hand into the splint, and then ease the fingers down into the warm mass of pellets, allowing the mass to ooze up between each finger. Make sure you have the fingers well-aligned. At this time, do not worry about adhering the finger separators to the finger pan. The goal now is to get adequate contouring, good contact with each finger, and proper alignment overall. Once you have achieved these goals, have the child remove his hand and quickly cool your finger separator portion with cold water or a commercially available cold contact spray (see How to Have a Second, Third, and Fourth Hand When You Really Don't section in Chapter 3).

Next, attach the pellet separators to the finger pan. Because the pellets are an elastic material, they will bond to any thermoplastic material from which you fabricate your hand splint. If your hand-splint material is coated with a non-stick surface, you first will need to remove the surface coat using a commercially available brush-on solvent or by scratching the coating off with the edge of a knife, scissor blade, or other sharp object. Use a heat gun to dry heat both surfaces, and then press them together. Additional spot heating around the edges of the pellet mass while pressing hard into the finger pan will ensure a strong bond.

Using these pellets as finger separators is especially beneficial for children with arthrogryposis because often every digit presents with a different deformity. The pellets enable the therapist to align each finger individually so that, regardless of its deformity, each finger has a customized alignment.

Another benefit of using these pellets is that they have 100% memory. If you make a mistake or do not get the proper alignment on the first attempt, toss the pellets back in the hot water and resoften them. If finger separators are necessary for a patient who is likely to "scrunch" the mass (such as an uncooperative child or one who demonstrates significantly increased muscle tone), you may prefer this pellet method over other materials that do not have memory. Because materials without memory cannot be reused or reshaped after they harden, using thermoplastic pellets is less wasteful and therefore, more cost effective. Using pellets to fabricate finger separators adds weight to the hand splint. Consider this factor before you select a material to use for separators. Keep in mind that additional weight is not always detrimental. If a child with ataxia is being splinted, having additional weight may be beneficial by inhibiting extraneous movements.

In the child with sensory modulation problems, the additional weight may increase proprioceptive feedback.

### Base for a weight-bearing splint

One of the most beneficial developmental outcomes of upper extremity weight-bearing is the proprioceptive input it provides and the support and maintenance of palmar arch development it offers. Many of the pediatric upper-extremity, weight-bearing splint patterns available are designed to keep the wrist in extension, but the pan on which the hand rests often is only a gross contour or mitt design. One way to achieve greater palmar contact is to fabricate the base of a weight-bearing splint from thermoplastic pellets. Place a large mass of softened pellets on a hard surface, which is covered with waxed paper or lightly greased with liquid soap or lotion. Next, place the child's hand in wrist extension, thumb abduction, and slight finger abduction. Quickly, before the softened mass of pellets starts to harden, depress the child's hand into the pellets. It is best if this is achieved with the child in a weight-bearing position. Quickly cool the mass while the hand is still in place. When the pellets have cooled sufficiently and you remove the child's hand, a perfect impression of the hand in a weight-bearing position will be left. Any excess can be trimmed away before the material is completely hardened (see Chapter 4 for fabrication instructions for the clamshell weight-bearing splint). For children who have flat palms and little evidence of arch development, you can create a slight arch using your finger to push up the material (before it completely cools) from under the base, thereby creating a subtle arch in the palm (Figure 2.1).

As the child grows, the same base can be reused by reheating the pellets and fabricating a new base whenever necessary. This makes the pellets a very cost-effective choice for a weight-bearing splint base.

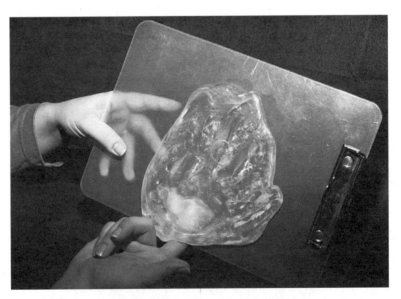

Figure **2.1** Creating a subtle palmar arch in the base of a weight-bearing splint

### Web opener under neoprene thumb-abduction splint

On occasion, a neoprene thumb-abduction splint is not sufficient to keep a child's thumb properly abducted for function. If muscle tone is moderately to severely increased, or significant soft-tissue constrictions are evident in the web space, neoprene may not be rigid enough to provide adequate thumb abduction and functional thumb opposition. Because the neoprene allows motion to occur, it is often the material of choice when fabricating a functional splint. One way to achieve more static and aggressive positioning, while still allowing some motion, is to use a combination of soft and hard splinting materials. To incorporate a static web opener into a neoprene thumb-abduction splint, soften a small mound of pellets and knead them together to form a mass. Next, conform the softened pellets into the child's web space while positioning the thumb in sufficient abduction to allow maximum opposition. The pellets should drape an equal distance around both the volar and dorsal surfaces (Figure 2.2). The finished product should be thick enough to rigidly maintain the desired thumb position but should not be bulky. Trim any excess material and allow the customized web opener to completely cool. Once hardened, place the web opener in the child's web space, and then put a neoprene thumb-abduction splint over it to hold it in place. The neoprene splint must fit snugly to hold the web opener in place but not so snugly that circulation is compromised.

### Palmar arch support under neoprene thumb-abduction splints

For children with poor palmar arch development, fabricating an arch support to be worn underneath a neoprene thumb-abduction splint is a nice option. This splint adaptation should be fabricated only if the child has limited thumb abduction in addition

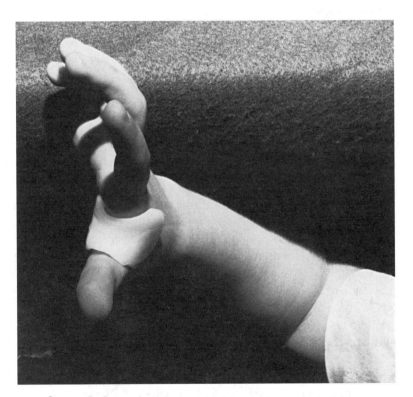

Figure **2.2** A web opener made from Adapt-It Thermoplastic Pellets

to poor arch development. If thumb abduction is sufficient, there are other palmar arch supports that can be fabricated without "over splinting" the thumb (Patterson, and Flanders, 1992). As in the above techniques, a mound of pellets is softened in hot water and then kneaded into a uniform mass. This mass of pellets is then conformed to the child's palm while the hand is held in an open position. Rather than allowing the material to harden in the passive, flattened shape of the child's palm, subtly create palmar arches by positioning the child's metacarpal bones in a slightly spherical position. Trim any excess material and allow the arch support to cool completely. The finished product, when worn under the modified neoprene thumb-abduction splint (with or without wrist component), will provide facilitory cues for arch development during functional and weight-bearing activities. If the arch support is well-conformed and the correct thickness, it should be tolerated comfortably underneath a neoprene splint and should be held snugly against the palm by the pressure the splint inherently provides. The reason that the *modified* neoprene thumb-abduction pattern should be used with the palmar arch support, versus the *standard* neoprene thumb-abduction pattern, is because it covers more of the palmar area. Therefore, it maintains contact with the entire arch support and holds it in the proper position.

### Thermoplastic rivets

Adapt-It Thermoplastic Pellets are an excellent material choice for fabricating your own rivets. By softening a small amount of pellets in hot water, tiny masses are formed that can then be rolled and flattened into rivets to make permanent strap attachments (see Chapter 3, Permanent Straps section, for further discussion and complete instructions).

## X-Lite (Hexcelite)

X-Lite is a low-temperature thermoplastic material with an open-weave design. It is available in rolls with 2-inch, 3-inch, 4-inch, or 6-inch widths. The material can be cut to size in its hardened form and then softened in hot (160°) water until pliable. The material is self-bonding. Therefore, the splint's rigidity can be increased easily by layering strips of material. X-Lite is easy to work with and has excellent memory. Because of its open-weave design, it is a nice material for hygiene splints because it allows air flow. Unfortunately, the benefit of this open-weave design also has a down side. The high percentage of perforations make this material slightly uncomfortable against the skin. For this reason, it is not the best material selection for a child with tactile defensiveness.

Because X-Lite is sold in strips and conforms so well, patterns often are not used when working with this material. Rather, an appropriately sized piece is placed against the patient's hand, elbow, fingers, etc., molded into the desired position, and held in place until cooled. Once hardened, the excess material easily can be trimmed to fit. Because all edges will be rough (due to the open weave), we recommend finishing the splint edges with Aquaplast Ultra Thin Edging Material. The open-weave design leaves the splint with little closed-surface area to adhere Velcro® for strapping. Peeling off the backing on self-adhesive Velcro and placing it against your X-Lite splint surface will rarely work. Dry heat the glue on the self-adhesive Velcro for 5–8 seconds with a heat gun and also spot heat the splint in the place your Velcro will attach. This way when the heated Velcro glue is placed against the heated X-Lite, a more stable bond is created. Some of the more common uses we have found to be especially helpful with pediatric splinting follow.

### Finger separators on pan of resting-hand splint

X-Lite can be used to fabricate finger separators on the pan of a resting-hand splint. Cut a strip of material so that it is the full length of the finger pan and about 1 1/2 times the width of the finger pan. The excess width is necessary in order to have sufficient material to form individual raised ridges between each finger (Figure 2.3). Usually, a single layer of X-Lite will provide adequate rigidity for finger separators. However, if necessary, two layers of material can be pressed together to increase the rigidity. If two layers are used, it is easiest to mold them simultaneously rather than individually. This is accomplished by firmly pressing the two heated pieces together prior to forming the finger separators. Once the separators have been formed and are hardened, they must be attached to the pan of the resting-hand splint.

If the hand splint was fabricated from an elastic material, a dry bond with a heat gun usually is sufficient to adhere the finger separators to the finger pan. However, the edges of the X-Lite must be aggressively smoothed into the finger pan to create a strong bond. If the hand splint was not fabricated from an elastic material, creating a strong attachment is more difficult. Because the X-Lite does not meld well into a rubber or plastic material, plastic finger rivets can be used to secure the finger separators to the pan of the hand splint. If rivets are unavailable or are uncomfortable for the client, the separators can be attached to the pan by using strips of Moleskin™ to tape down the X-Lite.

### Web opener

A web opener that can be worn alone or under a neoprene thumb-abduction splint can be made with X-Lite. Cut an oval piece of material, soften it in hot water, and then conform it to the child's web space while the thumb is maintained in adequate abduction. Allow the material to drape slightly over onto both the volar and dorsal surfaces (Figure 2.4). Trim any excess material and allow it to harden completely. If a single layer of material does not provide enough rigidity use an additional layer, but once again, it is easier to fabricate if both layers are adhered together prior to forming the web opener. When worn alone, a strap must be attached to the volar aspect, which then crosses across the palm, around the ulnar border of the wrist, and then across the dorsum of the hand to reattach to the dorsal aspect of the web opener. If worn under a neoprene thumb-abduction splint, the splint should provide adequate pressure against the web opener to maintain it in the correct position. Using X-Lite as a web opener underneath a neoprene thumb-abduction splint obviously is not as comfortable as an Adapt-It Thermoplastic Pellet or Putty Elastomer™ web opener. However, it is much lighter and offers slight aeration because of

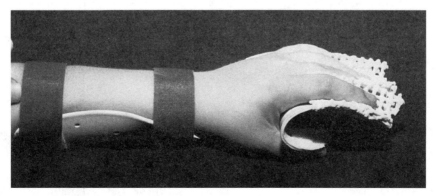

Figure **2.3**　Using X-Lite as finger separators on the pan of a resting-hand splint

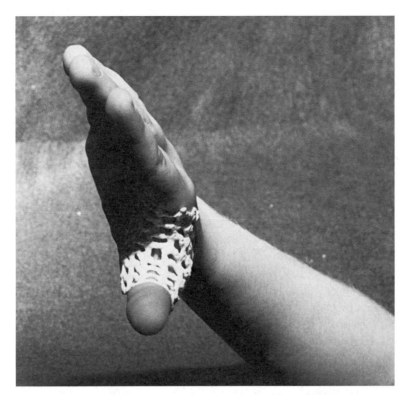

Figure **2.4** An X-Lite web opener can be worn under a neoprene thumb-abduction splint

its open-weave design. Take into consideration all these factors as well as the integrity of your client's sensory system before making a material selection for a web opener.

### Thumb spica

As mentioned above, pre-cut patterns are not always necessary when fabricating splints with X-Lite. Because of its superior ability to drape and conform, paired with its inherent memory, you can cut an appropriately sized piece of X-Lite (estimate how much is necessary to cover the area you are splinting) and mold it around your patient's thumb. If you feel a customized pattern is necessary, both the thumb spica and long thumb spica patterns and fabrication instructions using traditional thermoplastic materials can be found in Chapter 4. One easy modification of the long thumb spica is to shorten the proximal end of the pattern to make it a hand-based, rather than a forearm-based, splint. The advantages of fabricating these splints with X-Lite are the ease of fabrication, the open-weave design allowing for air flow, its light weight, and the ability to easily increase the amount of rigidity by layering the material. The disadvantage is that the material can be uncomfortable because of its texture and open-weave design.

### Circumferential finger or elbow splints (univalved)

Circumferential splint designs are easy to make with X-Lite because of the material's excellent ability to drape. Single or multiple layers of X-Lite can be cut and softened in hot water. Once pliable, the material is wrapped circumferentially around the extremity being splinted. The extremity must stay in the desired position while the X-Lite is cooling. Once completely cooled, a single, longitudinal cut can be made to univalve the splint for easy application and removal. For comfort, the edges will need to be smoothed or covered with Aquaplast Ultra Thin Edging Material. Although X-Lite is easy to drape, it is not necessarily the best material choice for a circumferential splint because of the material's texture. Also, the material's open-weave design, which, though advantageous for hygiene problems, can be irritating to the skin.

## Material Selection

When selecting a material, you first must consider what you want the material to accomplish. Do you need a material that drapes well and is rigid? Or is it most important that the material have good memory? As all materials cannot meet every demand, you must prioritize your patient's needs when considering which material is best suited for the splint you will be fabricating. The Materials Reference Chart (see Table 2.1 on page 36) can guide you through the selection process. In addition to these primary selection factors, other considerations to be taken into account are material thickness, color, solid versus perforated, and cost.

### Material Thickness

Low-temperature thermoplastics come in several thicknesses. They range from 1/16-inch to 3/32-inch, with 1/8-inch being standard. With pediatrics, 1/16-inch or 1/12-inch is commonly used to decrease the overall weight of the splint and to increase comfort and compliance. Thinner materials may also be selected for finger splints, arthritis conditions, and circumferential needs.

### Color

Having materials in an assortment of colors helps the therapist who primarily splints children. Unfortunately, not many products come in colors; white and beige continue to be standard. If you splint with elastics you have more of a selection because Aquaplast Watercolors™ and Prism come in bright, fun colors. Colors can make the splint more visually appealing and make it appear less medical, thereby making it more socially acceptable. A splint that is accepted by the child and the child's peers is more likely to be worn. A perfectly fabricated splint does not do any good if patient compliance is poor.

### Solid Versus Perforated

Many thermoplastics are available in both solid and perforated forms. There are advantages and disadvantages to both types. In general, solid materials tend to be more common and are available in more colors and thicknesses. Solid materials require less edge finishing, as there are no holes to cut through during pattern cutting that would make for rough, sharp edges. Solid materials can be more comfortable than perforated because the contact against the skin is more constant than the varying texture a perforated material provides. One advantage of perforated materials is that they allow for increased air circulation. If perspiration is an issue, perforations may be preferred. In addition, perforations tend to make a material less rigid, so it is often the best choice for a circumferential splint when the edges need to be pulled apart widely to allow donning and doffing of the splint. Pulling apart a solid material in this way is extremely difficult, and if it is a thick material, practically impossible.

## Soft Splinting Materials

As versatile as thermoplastic materials can be, a softer, more pliable material often is necessary. Common reasons for choosing a soft material over a thermoplastic may include poor skin integrity or skin sensitivity, weight, comfort, function, or to improve patient compliance. Following is an explanation of some commonly used soft splinting materials, but this list is by no means exhaustive. Use your creativity and imagination to explore other soft splinting options that may be effective for your patients.

### Neoprene

Neoprene is used extensively in pediatric splinting. Its high level of comfort leads to improved patient compliance, making splinting more effective. Neoprene can be purchased in a variety of thicknesses, colors, and textures. The different neoprene products on the market vary according to the amount of stretch the material allows, thickness, the material used for backing, texture, and, of course, color. When purchased commercially, neoprene is sold as either a sheet or a roll. The elastic neoprene material commonly is encased between a nylon lining on one side and a Velcro-sensitive pile on the other. Neoprene can also be purchased with a terry-cloth backing or with no material backing at all. Neoprene is available in thicknesses ranging from 1/16-inch to 3/8-inch. Products with the Velcro-sensitive pile on one side offer time-saving strap attachment because the backing allows for direct-hook Velcro attachment.

### Lycra

Lycra is an elastic-based material that recently has shown up in the literature and product catalogs as an alternative for soft splinting. The orientation of the material creates a circumferential dynamic force to the intended body parts to provide a correctional force. It has been said that Lycra controls abnormal tone, stabilizes posture, reduces involuntary movements, corrects alignment, and provides joint stability, thereby improving function in clients with neurological damage. The fabric is lightweight and porous and allows for increased comfort by the wearer. Full-body splints have been the primary use of Lycra to date. However, studies are under way using Lycra for upper-extremity splinting including a full-arm sleeve; gauntlet; and wrist, thumb, and glove splints (Blair, Ballantyne, Horsman, and Chauvel, 1995). Precautions to consider when using Lycra include skin breakdown due to perspiration or rash, circulation problems, and respiratory problems when the full-body suit is used.

### Elastomer

Elastomer is a silicone-based product designed to reduce hypertrophic scar formation. However, the use of elastomer has now expanded to include customizing splints for children. It is available in different forms and varying levels of firmness. There are liquid elastomers and putty elastomers. Liquid elastomers allow an easy working consistency for large surface areas, padding, or when a softer, less firm form is necessary. Putty elastomers, which we prefer because of the ease of use, range in consistency from soft to firm. To use a putty elastomer, rapidly knead equal amounts of elastomer putty and elastomer catalyst to create a uniform colored mass. Once the putty and the catalyst are joined, you have about 2 minutes of working time before the elastomer sets up. Once the elastomer is set it cannot be reshaped, so if you do not get your desired outcome on the first try, this is not a cost-effective material choice. In general, elastomer works well for curved or irregular areas, web space openers, and finger separators. In its hardened form, it is strong and resilient. It can be cleaned easily with soap and water and trimmed with scissors to obtain a precise fit without damaging the material. Some of the more common uses for elastomer, which are especially helpful with pediatric splinting, follow.

### Insert for small alignment changes

You have completed fabricating a hand-based splint for a pediatric client. The entire splint measures only 3 inches in length. When you place the splint on your client for a final check, you notice that while you were able to achieve optimal wrist extension, there is a slight ulnar deviation. If you attempt to reheat the wrist area to readjust the radial/ulnar alignment, you risk losing the perfect degree of wrist extension that you so painstakingly achieved. These small spot-heating modifications can be disastrous, especially on such a tiny splint. But a small amount of elastomer inserted inside the splint along the distal ulnar border can provide enough contact to "push" the hand toward the radial side until the desired alignment is achieved. This is often a more time-efficient way to make a small splint adjustment than reheating and reshaping the thermoplastic material.

### Finger separators in pan of resting-hand splint

Traditionally, finger separators have been constructed from individual finger loops made of strapping material. These can be time-consuming to fabricate and may require frequent maintenance and readjustment to maintain proper alignment. Elastomer can be used to form customized finger separators in the pan of a resting-hand splint. The technique used to fabricate the separators is similar to that used with the Adapt-It Thermoplastic Pellets. After completion of the resting-hand splint, a mass of kneaded putty is placed on the pan of the splint, and the patient's hand is placed in the splint, the fingers pressing down firmly into the mound of elastomer putty. You should have enough putty that when the hand is depressed into the mound, the excess naturally oozes up between the fingers to form ridges, which will serve as the separators. Be sure you have the desired finger alignment and maintain the fingers in this optimal position until the elastomer becomes firm. Remember, you have only 2 minutes of working time to knead the putty together, place it on the pan of the hand splint, and get your desired finger separator mold. Once the elastomer is firm, you can trim the edges so it fits into the pan of the splint. To bond elastomer to a thermoplastic material, elastomer adhesive works fairly well. Though it provides a secure attachment, it is not a permanent bond and can be torn off with a strong and sustained finger pull.

Because elastomer cannot be reused or reshaped once it hardens, it is obviously not an ideal material choice for finger separators for the child with spasticity or for an uncooperative patient who is at risk of "scrunching" the putty before it sets up, thereby making it useless. Because elastomer has no memory or ability to be reworked, if you do not achieve your ideal finger separators on the first try, you must start from scratch. In this situation, fabricating finger separators out of thermoplastic pellets would be a preferred method.

### Padding for comfort

Though not the most cost-effective choice, elastomer can be used to add a comfort pad if the child has an area that continues to have inappropriate redness or appears to be at risk for skin breakdown. Some children find an elastomer pad to be more comfortable than a foam pad. The elastomer certainly is more durable than foam padding. However, it is more difficult to attach to the underlying thermoplastic material.

### Palmar arch support under neoprene thumb-abduction splints

An elastomer insert can be fabricated to be worn underneath a modified neoprene thumb-abduction splint with or without a wrist component. The purpose of the insert is to provide support to the existing hand arches or to facilitate further development of arches. The inherent elastic properties of the neoprene hold the insert snugly in place against the palm. The modified thumb-abduction pattern must be used instead of the standard thumb-abduction pattern because the modified pattern covers more of the distal palmar area. This additional palmar coverage is necessary for the insert to stay securely in place and for appropriate contact to be made so the insert can put firm pressure against the palm, creating input into the hand arches.

### Increase pressure/contact for soft-tissue spreading

At times, a therapist wants to select an extremely conforming material to make good overall contact with the child's palm or other anatomical area. If the child demonstrates moderate to maximum increased muscle tone or is extremely uncooperative, the use of a highly drapable or conforming material (such as Polyform) is unrealistic. As any pediatric therapist knows, the softened material will be squished by the child and rendered unusable long before it can be adequately formed and allowed to harden. One way to compromise is to use a less-conforming material that is more user friendly (such as Ezeform) and fabricate a gross-positioning splint as desired. Next, to increase the skin-to-splint contact you sacrificed by not using a highly conforming material, use elastomer to "take up the slack" between the extremity and the splint surface. The better the contact is, the more likely you are to achieve soft-tissue spreading and optimal positioning. Another advantage of this method is that as the soft-tissue range improves, rather than fabricating an entirely new splint, you can redo your elastomer insert, which can then be replaced in your original gross-positioning splint.

### Elbow protectors

When a pad is needed to protect the elbow, elastomer can be a conforming and comfortable option. Often, patients with spinal cord injuries or other clinical conditions resulting in lower extremity paralysis will use their upper extremities to pull their bodies forward while prone, in a commando-crawl style. Due to the compromised sensory innervation, it is common for these patients unknowingly to cause friction injuries to their elbows. These injuries can become open, infected sores. To protect the elbows from this trauma, elbow protectors are a common solution. Elastomer putty can be used to fabricate an elbow protector that is held against the elbow when worn under a circumferential elbow sleeve. Because elastomer is durable and washable, topical antibacterial ointments can be placed on the open elbow sores, and the elastomer can be placed right over the ointment without damaging the elastomer or sticking to the underlying skin tissue.

### *Web space opener under neoprene thumb-abduction splint*

This is one of our favorite uses of elastomer. The technique used to fabricate a web space opener out of elastomer is similar to the technique for Adapt-It Thermoplastic Pellets. When a neoprene thumb abduction splint is not sufficient to keep a child's thumb properly abducted for function, an elastomer insert can provide the solution. Once the putty is kneaded together, the mass is conformed into the child's web space while positioning the thumb in sufficient abduction to allow maximum opposition (Figure 2.5). Before the putty hardens, allow a small amount of putty to drape onto both the volar and dorsal surfaces so that the web space is completely enclosed. Allow the elastomer to set up, and once it is firm, trim it as necessary. The finished product should be thick enough to maintain an open web space but thin enough to fit comfortably under the neoprene splint. The benefit of using elastomer as a web space opener insert rather than Adapt-It Thermoplastic Pellets is that the elastomer is more comfortable. It allows slight movement to occur as well, as it is not as rigid or static as the thermoplastic pellets. The disadvantage of using elastomer for a web space opener as compared to thermoplastic pellets is that elastomer has no memory, therefore, it cannot be reformed or reused once it sets up.

## Orthopedic Felt

Orthopedic felt is a non-stretchable material that can be used as a soft-splinting option when the client cannot tolerate hard thermoplastics. It is soft, but it is not conforming or firm. Orthopedic felt is most often used for circumferential elbow-extension splints

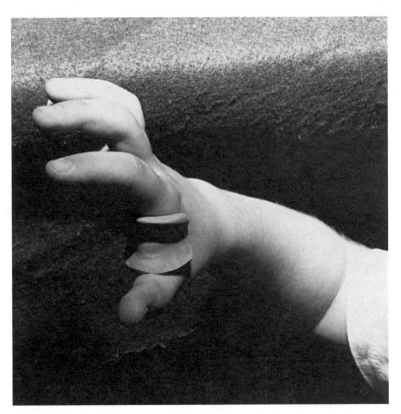

Figure **2.5** A web space opener made from elastomer can be comfortably worn under a neoprene thumb-abduction splint

or as palmar protectors for the severely involved hand. The felt is sold in sheets and is available in 1/8-inch, 1/4-inch, and 1/2-inch thicknesses. It is durable, washable, and absorbs perspiration, making it quite comfortable to wear.

## Polyurethane Foam

When a traditional thermoplastic material cannot be used for splinting because of fragile skin or pain, a high-density, fire-retardant polyurethane foam can be used to fabricate gross-positioning splints such as those for elbow flexion contractures. Foam is available in almost any width and comes in a variety of density levels. It can be purchased in bulk at large fabric stores or shops that sell foam for bedding and furniture construction. Cut the foam into a manageable size using an electric knife, which easily cuts through any density. This material has been used successfully to reduce significant limb contractures since 1978 (Anderson, Snow, Dorey, and Kabo, 1988). The benefits of using foam to splint the elbow are that it applies a uniform load, thereby preventing high-pressure areas from forming. The foam is also comfortable and provides neutral warmth, which may also help inhibit abnormal muscle tone (Farber, 1982). When polyurethane foam is used, you need to refabricate the splints using new foam at regular intervals because with constant use the foam softens and loses its firmness. When this occurs, it unfortunately also loses its ability to hold the extremity stable.

## Cloth Tape

Cloth tape, such as the kind used for first aid and sports injuries, can be used as an alternative material choice for infants. Multiple strips of cloth tape are layered upon each other to form a semi-rigid gross-positioning device for finger-, wrist-, or forearm-based splints for neonates. The tape is *not* circumferentially wrapped around the extremity. There is *no* contact of tape adhesive to the infant's skin. In the neonatal intensive care unit (NICU), this procedure could be used in lieu of neoprene or thermoplastics, which may be too heavy for some patients. Cloth tape is not durable, nor is it washable or conforming. However, it can be a cost-effective, lightweight option to provide gross alignment and positioning.

## Permagum

This silicone-rubber material is used traditionally by dentists to make dental impressions. However it is now also used to fabricate upper-extremity splints in the management of neonatal limb deformities and for children with neurological impairments. The authors who first reported the use of this material do not recommend it for older children, because the material is not rigid. For those interested in exploring Permagum's options further, refer to the article, "A New Material for Splinting Neonatal Limb Deformities" (Bell and Graham, 1995).

# Padding

There are a variety of splint padding materials available on the market. There are thin pads, thick pads, soft pads, firm pads, gel pads, adhesive pads and many others. If you do not need to pad your splint, don't. If you have spent a great deal of time trying to get a nice anatomical contour of your patient's palm, why throw padding on top of it and remove the benefit of the contouring? If you decide, however, that you do need padding in order to prevent skin breakdown, there are a few things to consider before making a selection. There are open-cell pads and closed-cell pads. Know which one you are purchasing. The advantage to closed-cell padding is that it is not destroyed by moisture. You can pre-pad your splint *prior* to heating it in hot water and forming it to your patient. This way the pad is already accommodated for and you do not have to think ahead and allow extra room in your splint for the pad. If you do pre-pad the splint, keep in mind that even though the padding is not compromised by contact with water, it will take about 2 hours before it dries and can be worn comfortably by the patient. You may want to select low-tack self-adhesive padding if you think it may be necessary to peel it off for readjustments. If it is not low tack, it is extremely difficult to remove neatly from the thermoplastic material. For stubborn pressure areas, we have found that gel padding such as Akton® padding or pressure-relief padding with a gel center work nicely.

Often, when therapists see a pressure area they add a pad to increase comfort and relieve pressure. What actually occurs, however, is that the padding adds *additional* pressure and exacerbates the problem rather than alleviating it. A better solution is to spot heat the problem area and remold it.

One splint that we do pad with regularity is the volar elbow-extension splint (see Chapter 4). When elbow flexion contractures are quite severe, the force of the muscles can create an intense high-pressure area at the distal and proximal points of the forearm. For this reason, this is the one design that we recommend you pad to increase comfort, thereby improving patient compliance with the prescribed wearing schedule.

## Strapping

Just as there are numerous types of padding materials on the market, there are numerous types of straps. While we usually don't have huge selections of padding available in our clinics, we do have several types of straps. When it comes to choosing a strap, most of the time we select standard 1-inch Velcro loop (colored, of course, because the kids will like their splints more) and mate it with standard white 1-inch self-adhesive Velcro hook. The standard Velcro is durable. We put the loop side next to the skin because the nylon side is not very comfortable. Depending on the splint you have fabricated, your strap may have a small or large amount of surface contact with your patient's hand.

With resting-hand splints, mitt splints, or anti-spasticity splints, we select a softer, more conforming strap to go across the MPs and the fingers. Several straps available today have a nice pile on one or both sides, which enables you to mate them with standard Velcro hook. Products like AlphaStrap®, Velcro Lo-Stretch Loop, and SoftStrap® are similar strapping products that are soft and comfortable and come in a variety of widths. Beta Pile II™ Loop comes in seven different colors. Neoprene and Neo-Plush are slightly stretchy and can also be used for straps. If you have a sewing machine available, webbing makes a nice strap, particularly for soft elbow-extension splints or when making a splint from orthopedic felt. There are other thick and sturdy products you can buy if you need strapping for an older child with severe spasticity.

Remember, you should not fabricate your splint so that all of the correctional or positioning forces come from the straps. If your patient is pulling out of the splint time and again, you should reconsider your splint choice. It is possible that you are asking for too drastic a change, but another possibility is that a different splint design is indicated.

You can purchase prefabricated straps if you wish. Some are available in a few different colors. However, they tend to be much longer than needed, and they are more expensive than buying standard Velcro loop by the roll.

For more ideas about straps and strapping options for those difficult-to-contain pediatric patients on your caseload, refer to the Anti-Houdini Fasteners section in Chapter 3.

# Practical Tips for Fabrication and Wear

Chapter **3**

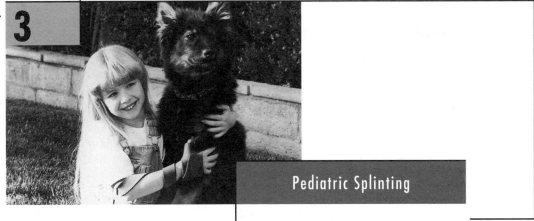

Pediatric Splinting

While a large portion of this book is dedicated to proper splint and material selection, we all know that the real challenge lies in proper fabrication. The more tricks of the trade a therapist is armed with, the better. With pediatric splinting the one thing you should always expect is the unexpected. You will continually need to make fabrication and splint modifications to ensure success. Several clinical challenges have given us the opportunity to use clinical reasoning and creative problem solving to find solutions to the variety of challenges that pediatric splinting creates. Learn to think on your feet and do not allow yourself to be boxed in to other people's recommendations (not even ours). Take what you know, add it to the information that follows, and then continue to keep an open mind and allow your own creativity to enable you to find solutions to the never-ending clinical problems you face each day. The following are suggestions we think you'll find helpful.

## How to Work with Neoprene

The benefits of splinting children with neoprene are well-known among therapists working in pediatrics. The material is comfortable for children to wear. It allows sensory input, and it enables children to grasp and move actively. It provides positioning and a passive stretch to the muscles. Its appearance is socially acceptable to children and their families. They like it!

Neoprene is readily available through most major distributors of splints and splinting materials. In addition to selling neoprene, most also sell Neo-Plush, which can be used interchangeably with neoprene. Neo-Plush has a soft texture to which Velcro hook mates nicely. The only drawback to Neo-Plush is that, to our knowledge, it only comes in beige. Neoprene, however, comes in over a dozen bright, fun colors, as well as a variety of types and thicknesses. Some therapists who live near a coastline might find that local scuba companies will donate their scraps. We have included a half dozen splints in our patterns that are made entirely or partially from neoprene. Because it is stretchy, neoprene adds a dynamic component to splints. It can also be used for straps. Neoprene conforms well, and because it comes in sheets you can make straps of any width you need.

Although neoprene is used commonly in pediatrics and it is rather simple to construct splints from it, there are a few secrets to working with neoprene that will make your neoprene splinting more successful.

## Cutting the Neoprene

Cutting patterns for neoprene takes planning. The patterns included in this book show that the pattern is drawn about 1/8-inch to 1/4-inch from the trace of the hand. This works well for splints made of a thin or standard neoprene, which is typically 1/8-inch to 3/16-inch thick. For some children this typical thickness of neoprene is not enough to control the spasticity in their extremities. For these kids you may need to select a material that is 1/4-inch thick. If you do, you will need to adjust your patient's pattern and draw it as much as 1/2-inch from the trace of the hand. Unless you make adjustments, your patient's thumb hole may be too tight. One of the easiest ways to avoid problems with the size of your splint is to make a pattern out of paper, tape it together and try it on your patient. Then, keep the pattern so that on the off chance the patient throws the splint out the car window on the way home (it's happened to us, it could happen to you), you will be able to make a new one easily. Do keep in mind, though, that neoprene stretches out after it has been worn a while. Sometimes it stretches substantially after just one or two months. That doesn't mean you have to refabricate it. If your initial purpose was to provide functional positioning for the hand, the splint may still do that, especially if the child has gained some active range of motion during first few months the splint was worn.

When you cut your neoprene pieces, you should cut your volar piece longer than your dorsal piece (Figure 3.1). When constructing your splint, the volar piece should be long enough to wrap across the palm, over the ulnar side of the hand, and onto the dorsum of the hand. If you are using standard Velcro hook-and-loop fasteners, attach a piece of 1-inch to 1 1/2-inch hook to the volar piece on the outside. Apply a 1-inch to 2-inch piece of the softer loop to the inside of the dorsal piece. (If you are using neoprene with a terry-cloth or pile backing, you do not need to add a piece of loop at all.) There are two main benefits to attaching the fasteners this way. First, when donning the splint, the dorsal piece will be pulled and placed over the hook on the volar piece. This creates force from the splint and pulls the child's thumb in the direction of extension. Second, as the child grows, the skin will have contact with the soft loop Velcro, which is much more

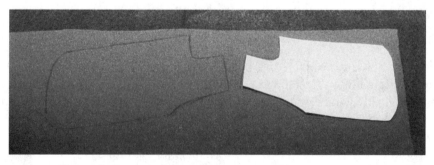

Figure **3.1**  Example of traced pattern pieces with volar piece longer than the dorsal piece

comfortable and tolerable than the scratchy hook. This will enable the child to wear the splint longer, assuming the neoprene has not become too stretched out and the splint still fits well at the web space.

## Constructing Splints Made of Neoprene

While some companies sell pre-fabricated pediatric neoprene splints, lots of therapists (ourselves included) still prefer to make a custom splint at their own clinics. It costs less, and it can be sent home with the child at the end of the day. The major objection we hear from therapists regarding making their own neoprene splints is the obligatory and time-consuming sewing that goes along with it. If you have a good industrial sewing machine available this is probably not a problem. But, even with a good machine it's difficult to keep the thread from catching on the Velcro hook and breaking. Although we admit there are certain circumstances in which sewing is unavoidable, we have spent a lot of time and energy investigating alternate methods. We finally came up with some pretty good "no sew" ways to attach neoprene to itself and attach Velcro fasteners to neoprene.

## Making Seams on Neoprene Splints

The best and fastest way we have found to make seams on our neoprene splints is to iron on Melco® tape (also referred to as neoprene tape). It is a thin, narrow nylon strip with a heat-activated adhesive on its underside. It comes in a variety of colors and is economical. The only sources we are aware of that sells it are the Benik Corporation and North Coast Medical. When the tape is used at a seam with an adhesive, the attachment is strong. Once the tape is applied and cooled, the splint can be cut or trimmed as needed directly over the seams. Cutting the tape will not cause it to lift or peel. The good news is that Melco tape is easy to apply to a splint with a straight seam such as the standard neoprene thumb-abduction splint. The not-so-good news is that it is trickier to apply to a curved seam such as the ones found in the modified neoprene thumb-abduction splints. Melco tape is applied using a standard household iron. In the directions below when we refer to a seam we mean the ends of two pieces of neoprene butted up against each other, not one piece overlapping another piece. If you have two seams to make, start with the most curved seam. You may find that using a few smaller pieces of tape is easier than one large piece. The pieces will adhere to each other if they overlap. If you do not get the hang of it the first time, don't give up—it really does work well.

## Directions for Attaching Melco Tape to Neoprene

1. Apply an adhesive of your choice to the ends of both pieces of neoprene. You can use Scotch™ Permanent Adhesive Glue Stick, Rubatex® cement, or any other neoprene glue (follow the product directions as indicated). Match up the two neoprene pieces.
2. Place the Melco tape over the seam.
3. Using a clothing iron set at a medium temperature, press down firmly, and apply pressure for about 10 seconds (Figure 3.2). *Do not slide the iron* or the tape will ball up. Use caution whenever ironing on neoprene as it tends to scorch easily.

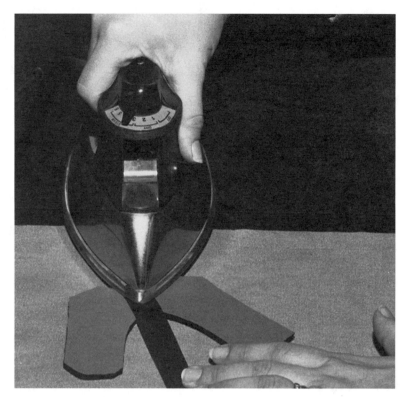

Figure **3.2** Ironing Melco tape onto neoprene over a seam

4. You will be able to peel the tape off when it is warm if you need to correct a mistake. Once the tape is cooled, it cannot be peeled off. When it is cool to the touch, test it to make sure that it has attached completely. If any of the edges lift up, repeat step 3.

5. To adhere the tape to curves such as the opening for the thumb, you need to place something cylindrical and solid into the hole (such as a dowel). Rock the iron back and forth over the tape for 10 seconds.

6. **Note:** If you are using neoprene with a pile or terry-cloth backing on the underside, you may be able to use a piece of Velcro hook temporarily to hold the two pieces of material together while you iron the Melco tape on the nylon side. Remove the hook after the tape has cooled (Figure 3.3).

## Attaching Velcro to Neoprene

While we haven't found a foolproof way to attach standard Velcro hook and loop to neoprene, we did find a type of Velcro that attaches to neoprene beautifully. Velcro 0143 hook-and-loop straps are heat-sensitive products that come with a pre-applied, heat-sensitive adhesive that can be ironed onto neoprene in about 2 minutes. The product is non-toxic, and it makes a bond that is as permanent as hand or machine sewing. This form of heat-sensitive Velcro is just recently being distributed by North Coast Medical. It can also be purchased directly from the Velcro USA Company (see Appendix B) or one of their distributors.

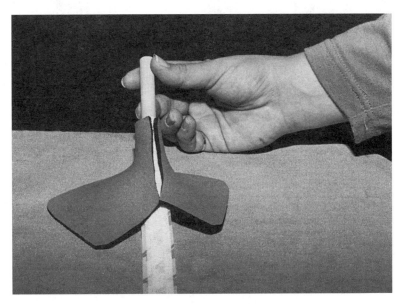

Figure **3.3**   Using Velcro hook to hold the pieces of neoprene together prior to ironing Melco tape over seam

## Directions for Attaching Heat-Activated Velcro (0143) to Neoprene

1.  Heat a clothing iron to the cotton setting. Use a dry iron. (Although the manufacturer says a steam iron can be used, a dry iron is working better in the clinic.)

2.  Cut a piece of hook or loop and round the edges. (Round edges do not pull off the material as easily as square edges, so this will make your strap even stronger.) Position the piece, adhesive side down, on the neoprene.

3.  Place a paper towel over the Velcro to prevent accidental melting of the materials.

4.  Press down for about 1 1/2 to 2 minutes, Move the iron around over the paper towel to avoid burning it. Check your materials frequently. Keep the iron off the neoprene itself as it tends to scorch. You can use the tip of your iron but don't use too much force or you might smash the Velcro hook.

5.  You will know your fastener is attached when you see a thin line of clear adhesive around the perimeter of the Velcro (Figure 3.4). Do not test (pull on) the strap until it is completely cool.

If you don't have Velcro 0143 at your clinic, there is one more ironing method you can try. There are some heavy-duty fusible webbing products available through cloth and fabric stores that you can use to attach Velcro to neoprene. Bonds using these products are not as permanent as the previous two we shared, but they work pretty well, and if they come off they can be ironed back on quickly.

Purchase a product like Aleene's® Ultra Hold Iron On Fusible Web™, available at most fabric or arts and crafts stores. Other brands that are heavy duty and have paper backing will also work, but you might have to play around with the manufacturer's directions before you get a good bond. We have tried heavy-duty hem webbings without paper backing, but they aren't able to take the heat of the iron for long. The thickness of the Velcro strap requires ironing for more time than most of the packages recommend, and

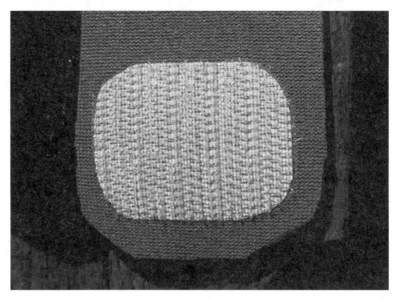

Figure **3.4**   Close-up showing glue along the perimeter of the
Velcro, indicating a secure bond

these hem webbing products seem to evaporate. The following directions are for attaching
a piece of standard Velcro loop, loop side down, to a piece of neoprene using Ultra Hold
Iron On Fusible Web. The texture on the loop side of the Velcro provides a good contact
for the fusible webbing. The slick nylon surface found on the back of the hook and loop
does not attach well with the webbing. But you can decorate or write the child's name
with fabric paints on the flat nylon side of the loop. If you attach the loop in the following
manner you will have to sew only the Velcro hook onto the splint.

### Directions for Attaching a Velcro Loop Strap to Neoprene Using Fusible Webbing

1. Heat a clothing iron to the cotton setting. Use a dry iron.
2. Cut your fusible webbing and paper backing to the shape of your strap, about 1/2 of
   the length. Round the edges of the strap and webbing. Trim the loop of the Velcro for
   better adhesion.
3. Place the fusible webbing (and the paper backing), rough side down on the neoprene
   where you want your strap to go.
4. Iron directly over the paper for *3 to 5 seconds only.* This will adhere the webbing
   slightly. The bond will be strong enough for you to remove the paper backing
   (Figure 3.5).
5. Place the strap, loop side down, directly over your webbing. Cover the strap with a
   paper towel to prevent glue from sticking to your iron. Iron the strap for roughly 30
   seconds (Figure 3.6). Check your strap every 15 seconds. While ironing, monitor the
   neoprene to make sure you are not scorching it.
6. Do not pull on the strap until it is completely cool.
7. For extra security, you can tack down the corners with needle and thread.

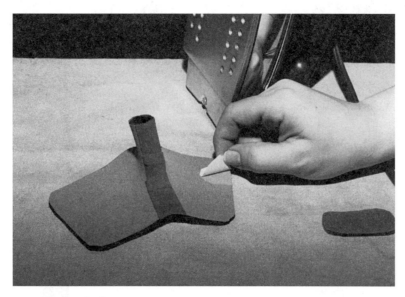

Figure **3.5**  After fusible webbing is adhered to neoprene, peel off paper backing

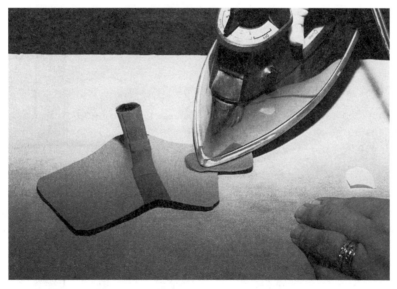

Figure **3.6**  Iron strap, loop side down, onto neoprene (paper omitted to demonstrate procedure)

## Using Neoprene as a Glove

There is one final benefit of neoprene worth discussing. We have already mentioned that neoprene does not inhibit sensory input or active movement completely, and it is very comfortable to wear. There are some occasions, however, when you want to select a splint that provides stronger positioning into opposition, or more support of the wrist or arches than you typically can achieve with a neoprene splint. The modified neoprene thumb-abduction splint and the modified neoprene thumb-abduction splint with wrist component serve as excellent splints under which you can insert a variety of positioning devices. Using materials such as elastomer and Adapt-It Thermoplastic Pellets, you can make a web opener or a palmar arch support to go under your patient's neoprene splint.

You can also use a scrap of thermoplastic material to construct an ulnar gutter to be worn at the wrist, under the splint, to help correct mild ulnar deviation. An ulnar gutter is a small square of thermoplastic material that conforms around the wrist joint (equal distance proximal and distal to the joint itself) and drapes from the middle of the dorsal surface of the forearm to the middle of the volar surface of the forearm. If you order a neoprene splint from Benik Corporation, they will add an aluminum stay and pocket for a small charge. This aluminum stay is slipped into the pocket on the volar surface to inhibit wrist flexion. If you are feeling *really* creative you can use some scraps of neoprene and construct a pocket using the Melco tape, into which you can place your own aluminum or thermoplastic stay. (We like making a stay out of elastic materials because they have 100% memory and can be reshaped if the child has changes in positioning and range.) If you prefer, you can use a thin piece of perforated material such as super perforated Aquaplast and sew directly through the perforations to the outside of the splint.

## Cleaning Neoprene

Because kids are kids, and because neoprene absorbs moisture like drool and sweat, neoprene splints need to be washed regularly. They can be washed gently in warm water with a mild soap. Rinse them well to eliminate any soapy residue, and use a towel to remove excess moisture. Neoprene splints should be air dried, never put in a clothes dryer. If you have added any thermoplastic or aluminum stays or other components, remember to remove them before washing.

## How to Make a Teeny-Tiny, Itsy-Bitsy Splint

Pattern making and splint fabrication are challenging enough on their own, but when you add the challenge of completing these same tasks for a tiny hand, splinting can become frustrating. The following are tips to help you fabricate splints on small hands.

Shrink larger patterns on a photocopier using the reducing feature, or if possible, place your patient's hand directly onto the copier and press the print key. Once you have a pattern that works well for a particular child, you can use this same suggestion to enlarge it by placing the pattern on the copier and pressing the enlarger button. This will help you refabricate the splint when necessary because of the child's growth. Using this technique does not allow you to have an exact customized splint pattern; however, there are times when you are not able to get the child's hand open adequately to get a precise pattern anyhow. This may occur with the more severely involved patient who has significantly increased muscle tone.

In such a situation it *is* acceptable to cheat. Therapists do not like to talk about this, but realistically, there are times when you have to break a few cardinal rules to fabricate an effective splint. If you were fortunate enough to have a splinting course in college, you probably had the opportunity to make only one or two splints. Both probably were fabricated on a totally compliant, neurologically intact lab partner. You learned *not* to use your fingertips but rather to grossly handle and cradle your heated material to prevent fingerprinting. You learned always to form the splint directly onto the patient so that your end product was *customized*.

These are good rules in theory, but theory is not always reality. With pediatric splinting, you really have no choice except to use your fingers. Splinting small children is an intricate task and our hands are just too big for some of the conforming and aligning that is necessary. If you attempt to complete 100% of your splint formation on the child's hand, you will inevitably run into problems. Initially, the material is too hot to place directly onto a child's sensitive skin. Once you do place it against their skin, you may still have 4 minutes working time before the material starts to firm up. What are the odds of getting a 2-year-old to hold an extremity in a precise position while holding still for 4 minutes? There is nothing wrong with completing partial fabrication on your own hand, on the patient's non-involved hand (when there is only hemiplegic involvement), on the hand of a similarly sized patient with less neurological involvement, or even on the hand of a sibling if the patient has one. The key is to get the partially firm splint onto the client's hand for final customization while the material still has some working time left. In this way, you can finalize size, alignment, arches, or any other custom fittings that need to be completed.

If this technique is used, you should assess the patient's hand first and create a visual picture in your mind of the optimum alignment as well as the maximum available range. When you are pre-forming the splint on yourself, a sibling, etc., try to duplicate this visual memory as closely as possible so that in the final forming stage on the client's hand only small changes need to be made.

Also, because small, intricate patterns and splints can be so difficult to make, keep any old splints and patterns in your clinic as prototypes. Then they are available to try on other patients for assessment or "trial" purposes.

One of the most frustrating experiences in pediatric splinting is when you have just completed a splint but need to make a minor adjustment. You don't dare get the splint near the heat gun for fear of meltdown, but the splint is so small that you are unable to submerge just an isolated spot in the hot water in the splint pan. In this situation, use a kitchen baster to draw up hot water from the splint pan. Then, slowly squeeze the baster bulb to run the hot water on the precise point you are attempting to spot heat for your small modification.

In review, here are suggestions for fabricating a teeny-tiny, itsy-bitsy splint:
- Reduce/enlarge patterns on photocopier.
- Use your fingers.
- Partially pre-form the splint on yourself, the patient's non-involved extremity, or a sibling's extremity.
- Save old splints and patterns.
- Use a kitchen baster to spot heat.

## How to Have a Second, Third, and Fourth Hand When You Really Don't

Not many of us have the luxury of having a certified occupational therapy assistant (COTA), physical therapy assistant (PTA), or therapy aide with us at all times. For those times when you really could use a second pair of hands but don't have them, read on.

If your clinic has a refrigerator, keep a strip of Thera-Band® in it at all times. When you are making a forearm-based splint, you can wrap the strip of cold Thera-Band around the forearm once you have placed the thermoplastic splint on the client. Not only will the Thera-Band hold the material in place proximally while you now are free to go distally for conforming and aligning, but the coldness will speed the cooling time.

A similar technique is to wrap the forearm portion of the splint with Coban® or an elastic bandage wrap to hold the material snugly so that both your hands are free to conform the wrist and hand portion. This method will leave a textured mark on the outside of the splint if using a plastic- or elastic-based material. Though it does not create any comfort problems for the child, it does affect the overall cosmetics of the splint and therefore may not be a preferred method.

Though sometimes it is nice to have a thermoplastic material with a long working time, this can be problematic when your biggest challenge is to get a child to sit still long enough to let the formed splint cool completely. For these times, commercially available products that quickly cool down your material can be lifesavers. There are two popular products, Cold Spray and Quik-Freeze®. Cold Spray has been around for years and most therapists are familiar with it. It contains hydrofluorocarbons, and it is flammable. Quik-Freeze is a newer product, and it has no hydrofluorocarbons or methyl chloroform, has low toxicity, and is non-flammable. Though Quik-Freeze may be more environmentally friendly, it also costs more than Cold Spray. When using Quik-Freeze, be sure to follow the manufacturer's directions. Do not spray directly onto the skin, as it can cause frostbite. Because of this contraindication, it obviously is not a good choice if using a perforated material unless you plan on removing the splint from the child's extremity before spraying it.

If you choose not to use a commercially available product, there are other low-tech ideas that can be used just as effectively as a canned cooling agent. Once you have the splint formed, you can quickly cool it by running the child's extremity (with the splint still on) under cold water. If a sink is not accessible, have a large tub of cold water sitting nearby and when the splint is completed, dunk the child's extremity into the tub. If these procedures are too alarming for the child, drape wet, cold washcloths over the splint. If the child has good function in the extremity that is not being splinted, you can fill a squirt gun with cold water and the child can squirt the splint to speed the cooling process.

One other simple tip is to splint in sections. This technique can be used with larger children when there is more material to handle at once. You can heat portions of the splint at a time so that fabrication takes place in stages, enabling you to form smaller, more manageable sections.

There are some elastics that temporarily bond together when heated but when cooled easily pop apart. This quality can be put to use if you need an extra pair of hands because it enables you to bond two edges together so that the material does not drape uncontrollably. Then your attention can turn elsewhere to conform and align as needed (Figure 3.7). This works especially well for circumferential and elbow-extension splints.

Another way to feel like you have an extra pair of hands is to use gravity to your advantage whenever possible. Remember that gravity is a very strong force and when given the opportunity, it will either assist us or resist us. Unfortunately, there are times when we know that gravity is resisting us, but we have no choice except to splint in a

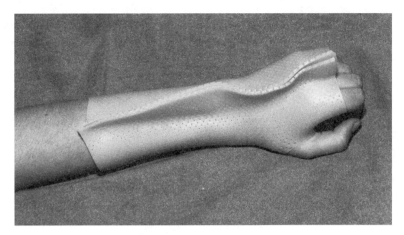

Figure **3.7** Precise positioning and conforming can be achieved while the splint is held in place with a temporary band created by lightly pinching the edges together

particular position. An example of this is when you are fabricating a volar, forearm-based splint while your patient is sitting upright with the forearm in a pronated position. Gravity or not, if the splint you are fabricating is a forearm-based splint, you must fabricate it in the position that the splint will be worn. If you fabricate a resting-hand splint (worn with the forearm *pronated*) with the forearm in a *supinated* position, when the client dons the splint the forearm portion will not fit correctly. This is only a problem with forearm-based splints because of the rotation component of the forearm.

In review, here are suggestions for how to have a second, third, and fourth hand:

- Wrap forearm portion with refrigerated Thera-Band.
- Wrap forearm portion with Coban, Co-Wrap or an elastic bandage.
- Use Cold Spray or Quik-Freeze.
- Use a container of cold water; cold, wet washcloths; or cold water in a squirt gun.
- Splint in sections.
- Temporarily bond edges of elastics.
- Use gravity to your advantage.

## Anti-Houdini Fasteners

Although we would like kids to be independent with donning and doffing their splints, we do not want them to remove their splints at inappropriate times. No matter how much Velcro you use and how creative your strapping is, there are some children who are just born Houdinis. We have found a few anti-Houdini straps, which so far appear to be containing even the most difficult cases.

The use of Poly-Lock™ or Dual Lock® mated with standard loop Velcro results in a high-retention attachment. To understand how strong this attachment is, consider this comparison. The closure strength of standard Velcro hook to loop for lengthwise peel is 1 pound per square inch. The closure strength of Poly-Lock to standard loop is 25 pounds per square inch. The problem with using this fastener method is that not only is it difficult for children to pull a loop Velcro strap off Dual Lock or Poly-Lock, but it is also difficult for the caregivers. This bond is so strong that it really could be considered a permanent strap, although with effort, it can be separated. When this method is used, keep in mind that the loop Velcro will require more frequent replacement because the Poly-Lock wears out the loop pile quickly. Also, make sure the Poly-Lock is adhered well to the thermoplastic or it may pull off the splint during repeated openings and closures.

Another method is to use shoelaces in lieu of Velcro straps. This works best for circumferential splints but can also be used on any splint as long as the shoelace contact on the underlying skin is not uncomfortable or creating any problems such as circulatory or skin sensitivity. To use this strapping method, punch holes into both edges of the splint using a revolving hole punch (available through catalogs and leather and hobby shops). Then lace a shoelace through the holes for the entire length of the splint, just as you would lace up a shoe. A bow can be tied at the end to hold the lacing secure. If the child has adequate dexterity to unlace the shoelace, pull apart the two splint edges, and slip the extremity out, you can prevent the ability to unlace the shoelace by placing a shoelace keeper on the bow (Figure 3.8). Shoelace keepers are available at drug stores, shoe stores, and children's department stores. They come in several styles and characters, and usually are well received by children. Be selective when you buy shoelace keepers. Some are boxes designed to hold only infant-sized shoelaces and do not allow adequate room for larger-sized laces. We like the types that have a pliable elastic rubberband, which can accommodate a shoelace of any length, or those that open and clamp onto the shoelace.

Plastic diaper clips also can be used to fasten splints when you want to make it a little more difficult for children to remove splints by themselves. A diaper clip can be used on a piece of strapping that overlaps onto itself. For example, if you use a Beta Pile™ or other strap on the forearm portion of a wrist cock-up splint, make a slit on the side of the splint parallel to the edges of the splint. Put the strap through the slit from the inside to the outside and then back over itself. The diaper clip opens and clamps onto the strap (Figure 3.9).

An old-fashioned hook-and-eye attachment from a fabric store works quite well for neoprene splint closures. While it is possible to unhook a hook-and-eye with only one hand, it is not easy. It requires precise fine-motor skills. By hand-sewing a hook attachment to one side of a neoprene splint and the eye attachment to the opposite side, you create a closure as secure as Velcro but difficult to unhook with only one hand.

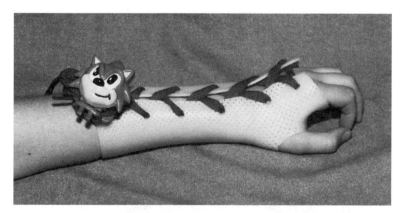

Figure **3.8** A shoelace and shoelace keeper serve as an excellent anti-Houdini fastener

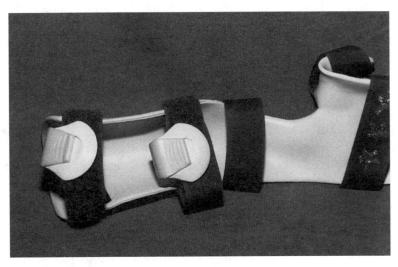

Figure **3.9** Plastic diaper clips secure the Velcro straps, making splint removal difficult

Another good choice for your little Houdini is metal safety buckles or safety webbing buckles. These buckles work on webbing and standard Velcro loop. They have a protective sheath that "locks" over the teeth of the buckle and keeps the skin safe from injury. These buckles require some degree of fine motor skill and are difficult for young fingers to unfasten by themselves.

You also can choose to use a metal lamp or ceiling fan pull chain, which is sewn directly over a Velcro or webbing closure (Allen, Flegle, and Watson, 1992). The trick is to allow only enough length to open and close the pull chain with slight tension and not to allow any slack in the chain. This way, it will require two hands to hook and unhook the chain. The chain alone would not be comfortable against the skin so make sure to sew it directly to the surface of the strapping material you select.

Although we have not personally used this method, a small luggage or diary lock also can be used to actually "lock" the splint onto the child. Because of its small size, it does not provide a lot of additional weight but potentially could be uncomfortable for some children because these locks are metal. The caregiver wears the key on a chain around the neck or keeps it in some other safe and accessible place (make sure to have a duplicate key). As you can imagine, this method may be controversial and not well-accepted by some parents. Be sure to use this method as a last resort and discuss other options with the caregivers before deciding on this more drastic method.

In review, here are suggestions for Anti-Houdini fasteners:
- Poly-Lock or Dual Lock mated with loop Velcro
- Shoelace strapping
- Shoelace keeper
- Diaper clip
- Hook-and-eye fastener
- Metal buckles
- Pull chain fastener
- Small luggage lock

## Permanent Straps

Having correct strap placement is critical for many splints to be effective. The more people involved in the care of your patient, the greater the chance the splint straps will be positioned incorrectly. When a child is in a residential care placement or in a classroom with several aides, there may be a dozen people responsible for donning and doffing the child's splint. It can be a challenge to instruct a number of caregivers, monitor their consistency, and follow through with the splint application. One way to increase the odds of the straps being placed correctly is to adhere one side permanently so the strap cannot be placed incorrectly. There are several methods you can use to attach one side permanently.

Traditionally, using rivets has been a common technique to attach a strap permanently to a splint. Because of the number of pieces and the tools required to fasten regular metal rivets, we often do not use them. Finger rivets (available from Rehabilitation Division, Smith and Nephew, Inc.) are easy-to-use plastic rivets. They are available in small and large sizes, and 100 rivets (50 sets) can be purchased for a reasonable price. Once you have punched an adequately sized hole into the thermoplastic and the strapping material, the rivets snap together easily by hand. Once snapped together, they are difficult (if not impossible) to pull apart. The small size works nicely to attach a strap to a thermoplastic splint. These rivets work best with 1/8-inch material thickness. When thinner materials are used, a gap remains between the rivet and the material when fully closed, and the rivet still has a 1/4-inch space (Figure 3.10). There are other plastic rivets available, such as Rapid Rivets (available from Sammons Preston), that can be changed and reused; these require a screwdriver to fasten and unfasten.

A more cost-effective way to attach a strap permanently to a thermoplastic material is to fabricate your own thermoplastic rivets out of scraps. The scrap thermoplastic should be a material that conforms easily such as a plastic (Polyform works well) or an elastic (such as Aquaplast). In addition to these scrap thermoplastics, Adapt-It Thermoplastic Pellets work especially well for this method. Once you have determined where you are

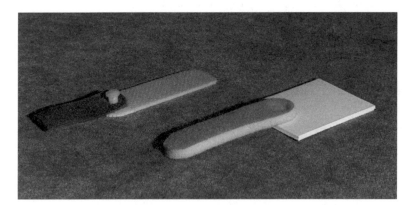

Figure **3.10** On the left, a small finger rivet is used to secure a thin strap to a thin piece of thermoplastic material, resulting in the rivet protruding from the splint; on the right a 1/8-inch piece of thermoplastic is secured to a thicker strap, leaving the rivet flush to the surface

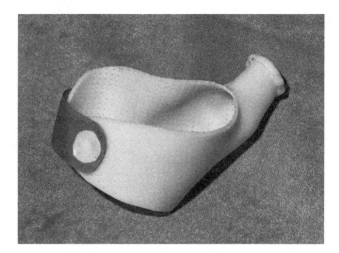

Figure **3.11**  A custom rivet made from Adapt-It Thermoplastic Pellets

going to place the strap, use a revolving hole punch to punch a hole through both your thermoplastic splint and your selected strapping material and line up the two holes. Rather than having two separate pieces that snap together, as in the finger rivet method, with this method you take only one pea-sized piece of heated material and roll it into a miniature hot-dog shape. Next, place this piece through both holes and quickly push the heated material into the strap on the one side and into the splint on the other side. Be sure to smooth the rivet flat so it will be comfortable against the child's skin (Figure 3.11).

Another technique to create a permanent strap is to directly bond a loop Velcro material, loop down, into the thermoplastic. This technique will work only with splints made of elastics or plastics because they have a "gooey" characteristic that allows the pile on the loop to "ooze" into the material, thereby creating a solid bond. First, use a heat gun to spot heat the splint in the exact spot you have identified for strap placement. Once well heated, quickly place the strap, with the loop side against the thermoplastic, and press it firmly into the heated material. Allow it to cool completely. One additional tip is to round off the edges of the Velcro loop before adhering it to the splint to prevent the strap from being pulled off. If you need to remove the strap, you must reheat the thermoplastic with a heat gun and once warm, peel the loop strap away from the splint.

As discussed in the Anti-Houdini Fasteners section, Poly-Lock or Dual Lock, when mated to Velcro loop, are such strong attachments that they also can be considered a permanent strap. Use this method on one side of the strap and standard Velcro hook and loop on the other side.

In review, here are suggestions for permanent straps:
- Finger rivets, Rapid Rivets
- Thermoplastic rivets
- Heat-bond loop Velcro directly into thermoplastic
- Poly-Lock or Dual Lock

## Miscellaneous Tips

When making splint patterns, use industrial paper towels instead of notebook paper. Paper towels, such as the kind found in most public restrooms, are made of strong paper but are not stiff and can be wrapped around the child's extremity to check for proper fit before tracing the final pattern onto the thermoplastic or other splinting material.

Keep a large number of splint patterns on hand in your clinic. Because paper eventually will wrinkle, tear, and become worn, you can trace preferred patterns onto exposed X-ray film, cardboard, or Naugahyde to create durable patterns that can be used over and over again. Naugahyde works especially well because it is pliable, and the pattern can be tried on the child to assess for fit prior to cutting.

If a child has a bony prominence that appears to be a potential source for a pressure area, you can use therapy putty to pre-pad the bony prominence prior to splinting (Figure 3.12). Because the putty softens with heat, you should use a putty of medium or firm consistency that will maintain its form even when a heated piece of thermoplastic is placed over it. When an area is pre-padded in this way, it creates a built in "bubble" to protect the potentially painful spot. Once the splint is completely cooled, the putty can be peeled off. If you are pre-padding with putty under a perforated material, you may find that some of the putty gets embedded in the holes. You can easily get the putty out by firmly pressing a mound of putty into the perforations of the cooled material, thereby pulling the excess out of the perforations. If this method does not remove all the excess, you can always use the trusty "poke with a paper clip" method.

When fabricating a forearm-based splint, flare the proximal edge of the splint away from the child's skin. If the splint edge is not flared away, it will rub against the skin and put pressure on the underlying muscle tissue, causing an uncomfortable and potentially dangerous situation for the child. When fabricating an elbow splint, flare both the distal and proximal edges (see Figure 4.58 on page 143).

When using elastic or other tacky materials, add a tablespoon of liquid soap or shampoo to the hot water before placing your thermoplastic material in it. Do not use a soap that claims to "cut grease" or has "lemon added" as these do not create the slick barrier necessary to prevent the material from sticking to itself. Soap decreases the amount of tackiness, but it does not eliminate it altogether so you still must take care to prevent tacky materials from touching. As much as we love Orfit, there are times when you end

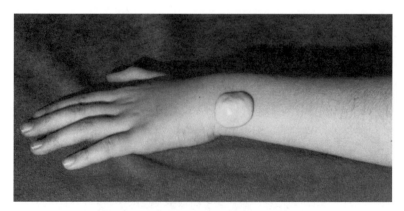

Figure **3.12**   Therapy putty can be used to pre-pad a bony prominence prior to splinting

up with a "glob" of material that cannot be "unglobbed." (It is a minor drawback to an otherwise versatile, useful material.) If your material tends to stick together even when you are putting soap in the water, make sure you are heating your thermoplastic at the water temperature recommended by the manufacturer. Using water that is too hot will create tackiness in some materials.

When tracing a pattern onto a thermoplastic material, we find that a colored grease pencil works well. It does not break like pencil lead, and it is not permanent like an ink pen. The grease pencil glides onto the thermoplastic material easily and makes a clear pattern line even on perforated materials. Because grease pencil is difficult to remove from thermoplastics, once the pattern is drawn, we recommend cutting just *inside* the grease pencil mark. In this way, the finished product will be free of markings, thereby improving overall cosmetics of your splint. Grease pencil marks can be partially removed by firmly rubbing with a soft, dry cloth or by using rubbing alcohol. However, both of these removal methods work best *before* the material has been heated. Once the material has been heated, the grease tends to embed in the thermoplastic and becomes harder to remove. Another technique used for pattern tracing is to use a scratch awl to transfer your pattern onto a thermoplastic material. This technique works, but you must scratch a deep groove in order to still see it on the material once it has been heated. This awl technique does not work well when using perforated materials.

Another miscellaneous tip is to cool your heat gun for 1 minute before shutting it off. By placing it on "cool" mode for this period of time, you will increase the life of your heat gun tremendously.

When attaching self-adhesive Velcro, Poly-Lock, or Dual Lock to a thermoplastic material, first peel off the paper backing and then dry heat the adhesive by holding it over a heat gun for 5–8 seconds. This will give you a much stronger bond when you press the adhesive into the thermoplastic. Be sure to use tongs or scissor-tips to hold the Velcro over the heat gun so you do not burn your fingertips.

Pediatric patients with physical disabilities frequently need a variety of medical and adaptive equipment to make their activities of daily living and mobility easier. Traditionally, splints have added to this "medical" look. Now, with colored splinting materials on the market, splints can look more pediatric and less medical. If colored materials are not an option due to budget constraints or because they are not available for the material you have selected, there are still other options. Using colored straps, you easily create a more pediatric-looking splint. It is not necessary to buy colored hook, as this portion of the strap is covered by the loop portion anyhow.

To further make your splint more fun to wear, use colored markers to draw on the splint. Non-toxic, permanent splint markers are available from Sammons Preston. These markers can be used to label or decorate the splint *prior* to heating the material. This way you can draw a design while the material still is flattened rather than after it is completed and may have curves that make drawing a challenge. If you are not artistically inclined, purchase carbon paper and a children's coloring book. Trace firmly over a selected picture (with the carbon paper underneath) and the design will transfer directly onto the splint pattern. Whenever possible, allow children to draw their own pictures or write their own names. This makes them part of the splinting process. Allow the markers to dry for about 30 minutes before placing the splint in hot water to prevent any running of the marker dye. If having this gap in time is inconvenient, the child could decorate the splint one day as part of the therapy activities, and the splint could be fabricated at the next therapy session. You also can decorate thermoplastic splints with stickers, rub-on tattoos, or decorations made from scraps of colored thermoplastic materials. (Adhere thermoplastic pieces together with dry heat for a secure attachment.) Neoprene splints can be decorated with non-toxic fabric paints or by using contrasting colors of neoprene tape (Melco tape) over the splint seams. This tape can also be used to make racing stripes or other decorative patterns. For those with a flair for fashion, why not sew a small strip of lace around the wrist? Any decoration that makes a splint more cosmetically appealing is likely to increase the child's acceptance of it and therefore, improve wearing compliance.

Depending on the size of the splint you are fabricating, it may be impossible to use your fingers to smooth all edges. If you have made a wrist cock-up splint with a thumb hole for a small child, your finger may be too large to place into the thumb hole opening to smooth the edges and prevent skin discomfort. For this reason, we like to keep several wooden dowels of varying widths in the clinic. These can easily be placed through any size opening and can be used to form or smooth those portions of the splint that are too intricate for your fingers. Dowels are inexpensive and can be purchased at most fabric, craft, and hardware stores. Dowels also can be placed through the thumb opening of a neoprene thumb abduction splint to provide a hard, stable surface to press against when ironing neoprene tape onto the thumb seam (see Figure 3.3 on page 55).

One of the most challenging situations in pediatric splinting is when you need to fabricate a hand splint for a child who has increased or fluctuating muscle tone or a child that is uncooperative. We have all had the experience of placing heated material against the child's hand in preparation for fabricating the splint only to have the child close their hand and "scrunch" the heated material. If you're splinting with elastics, this scenario is bothersome but not unmanageable as you can throw your scrunched material back in the hot water and it will go back to its original shape. If, however, you are splinting with a plastic material (which is a good choice for a spastic hand due to its rigidity), you do not usually have the luxury of a second chance. Once this material has been "scrunched," it may be unusable. One tip to help decrease the effects of what we call the "scrunch factor" is to pre-pad the splint with a low tack Polycushion® material. If you use a closed cell padding, you can attach it directly to your splint before you toss it in the water to heat it. Once the thermoplastic material with the Polycushion padding is removed from the water, the cushion serves as a buffer when you place it against the child's hand for fabrication. Now when the child's hand starts to close, the Polycushion absorbs the initial momentum and does not allow the fingertips to sink into the material. Obviously, it does not completely stop the "scrunch" but it does slow it down, which can make fabrication easier. If you do not want the splint to be lined, you can remove the Polycushion by peeling it off once the splint is completely cooled. You must use a padding with a low-tack adhesive backing or the cushion will not peel off well. If any remaining adhesive or cushion material stays on the splint, you can use Goo Gone® or a similar product to remove the remnants.

In review, here are miscellaneous fabrication tips:
- Make single-use patterns out of industrial paper towels.
- Make prototype patterns out of exposed X-ray film, cardboard, or Naugahyde.
- Pre-pad bony prominences with therapy putty.
- Flare the distal and proximal borders of the splint to increase comfort.
- Add liquid soap to water in the splint pan and use recommended water temperature.
- Use a grease pencil or scratch awl to trace patterns onto thermoplastics.

- Cool down heat gun for 1 minute before turning it off.
- Dry heat adhesive backing on Velcro before attaching to thermoplastic.
- Use colored thermoplastics, colored strapping, and permanent colored markers to improve cosmetics.
- Decorate splints with stickers, tattoos, scrap thermoplastics, fabric paints, neoprene tape, lace, etc.
- Use varying sizes of wooden dowels for thumb hole and spot fabrication.
- Pre-pad thermoplastic with low-tack Polycushion to decrease the "scrunch factor."

## Assessing Proper Fit

You have worked hard to fabricate a complicated splint. The finished product is beautiful. But even the perfect splint will not benefit the child if it is not worn. One way to improve patient compliance is to make sure the splint fits well and is comfortable. Once the initial fabrication is completed, ask yourself these questions to guide your assessment of splint fit and comfort:

Is the splint meeting its intended goal?

Is it maintaining the extremity in optimal alignment?

Is it supporting or stabilizing the intended joints?

Is the splint crossing any joint(s) other than the joint(s) it is intended for and thereby needlessly immobilizing a joint(s)?

Is the splint allowing the maximum mobility and function available to this child?

Is the splint maintaining natural palmar arches, while at the same time not "flattening out" the thenar eminence?

Are the palm and volar digital surfaces as open as possible, allowing maximum sensory experiences?

Are there any blanched areas on the skin?

Are there any red areas on the skin that do not disappear within 20 minutes of splint removal?

Is the forearm trough two-thirds the length of the forearm?

Does the splint respect the inherent anatomical dual obliquity of the hand?

Are all bony prominences free from pressure?

If the goal is to improve range of motion, is the intended joint positioned in submaximum range?

Is padding necessary or will added padding just increase pressure?

Are all edges smooth to the touch?

Does the splint require a lining to absorb perspiration?

Are all existing rivets, straps, or attachments free of rough or sharp edges?

Although a potential problem can be evident anywhere in the splinted extremity, there are certain areas that appear to be more prone to pressure areas. Dorsally, these include the MP joints of the hand and the ulnar styloid at the wrist. Because the volar surface anatomically has more natural padding, it is not as susceptible to pressure areas. However, one area to pay particular attention to on the volar surface is the MP joint of the thumb. In addition, the radial border of the wrist (styloid process of the radius) is vulnerable to pressure when a forearm-based splint is worn, especially if the wrist tends to be in ulnar deviation. When fabricating an elbow splint, the areas to monitor closely include the olecranon process of the ulna (which forms the point of the elbow) and the medial and lateral humeral epicondyles (the pronounced prominences of the elbow).

## Splint Wearing Schedules

For a splint to be successful, you must develop an appropriate wearing schedule for the child and caregiver to follow. The world's most perfect splint does not do any good if it is not worn appropriately. Wearing schedules vary and should be determined by taking into consideration the child's level of tolerance for the splint, the child's daily routine/schedule, and the purpose of the splint. The purpose of the splint will either be for 1) function, 2) hygiene, 3) protection/behavior, or 4) positioning.

Though schedules will vary according to individual needs, the following guidelines should be considered when determining the child's splint wearing schedule.

### Function

If the splint's purpose is for improved function, it is to be worn only during the day when the child is engaged in alert and active environmental exploration or a specific functional activity for which the splint serves as an adjunct.

### Hygiene

If the splint is for hygiene purposes, it can be worn up to 23 hours per day to maintain the integrity of the skin and underlying tissue.

### Protection/Behavior

If the splint's purpose is for protection/behavior, it should be worn during waking hours when the non-desired behavior is being demonstrated or is likely to be demonstrated.

### Positioning

If the purpose of the splint is positioning, the wearing schedule can be more difficult to determine. Referring back to the Splint Selection Flow Chart in Chapter One on page 20, ask yourself the following guiding questions to determine the most appropriate wearing schedule for positioning splints.

*Are you positioning the extremity to support a joint?* If this is the purpose, the splint should be worn only when the extremity needs support. This may be only while the patient is awake and active and the joint is likely to be malaligned due to influence of gravity, muscle weakness, or an imbalance in muscle action. If, however, the joint is also at risk for malalignment or other problems even when the child is at rest, then the splint wearing schedule should extend to night/nap wear. With children, it is a good idea to have the parents observe the resting position of the joint or joints in question while the child is sleeping. After the parent describes the resting position, you can better determine if proper alignment is being maintained or if the splint needs to be worn at night.

*Are you providing a splint to rest a joint?* A splint for this purpose is likely to be worn when inflammation is present, and the joint needs to be immobilized to allow rest and prevent further inflammation. This type of splint may be worn as much as possible both day and night, but its intended use is short-term or just until the inflammation subsides.

*Are you providing a splint to increase range of motion?* Positioning to regain lost range of motion seems to be the most subjective area in regards to wearing schedules.

There are several studies that provide us with more than enough information to confidently guide our clinical reasoning to determine appropriate wearing schedules. A discussion of the literature that will assist therapists with their clinical reasoning in this area follows.

The cause of limited range of motion falls into one of two categories: nonstructural changes and structural changes (McClure and Flowers, 1992). Nonstructural changes in periarticular tissues (tissues surrounding the joint) include pain and "protective" muscle contractions that, over time, lead to limited range of motion. Structural changes in periatricular tissues include shortening of joint capsule, ligament, muscle, or adhesions resulting from a combination of trauma and immobilization. The tissue undergoes compositional and structural changes such as extracellular water loss, glycoaminoglycan depletion, excessive collagen cross-linking, and fibrofatty deposition. These changes play a major role in the joint contracture process and ultimately limit passive range of motion. Regardless of whether the cause is nonstructural or structural in nature, the end result is shortened tissues, which then present clinically as a loss of range of motion.

It may be helpful to understand why tissue shortens. There are several different theories as to why this occurs. These theories are nicely summarized in the article "The Use of Splints in the Treatment of Joint Stiffness: Biologic Rationale and an Algorithm for Making Clinical Decisions" (McClure, Blackburn, and Dusold, 1994). One theory states that when collagenous tissues are immobilized in a shortened position, predictable changes occur.

These predictable changes include a decrease in the amount of collagen, glycosaminoglycons, and water. These decreased amounts are what biologically cause the tissue to become shorter and weaker. At the same time, this immobilization allows new intermolecular and intramolecular cross-links to be formed within the periarticular connective tissues in this new shortened state, which limits tissue extensibility.

A second theory states that the connective tissues shorten through a process of contraction. Some studies report that actin, which is a contractile protein, has been identified in fibroblasts and is responsible for ligament contraction. Others, however, believe that myofibroblasts, which are cells that resemble smooth muscle cells, may be the primary causal factor of connective tissue contraction (McClure, et al., 1994).

There is another theory that states that the cause of tissue shortening is related to adhesion formation. This process occurs when scar tissue forms between tissues that normally move relative to one another. These adhesions limit the tissue extensibility and lead to limited range of motion.

Regardless of the actual mechanism that causes tissue to shorten, the result of joint immobilization is a decrease in the functional length of the periarticular connective tissues and associated muscles that have been held in this shortened position. This decrease in length equals limited range of motion. The muscle then accommodates to this shortened immobilized position through biological changes that take place such as a loss in the number of sarcomeres.

Once the limitation in range has occurred, what kind of influence can our splints have on regaining the lost range? In theory, when the normal level of tissue strain is exceeded, biological changes occur. The capability of shortened tissues to undergo structural lengthening has been demonstrated in both basic science and clinical research. Collagenous tissues respond to increased tensile loading by increasing synthesis of collagen and other extracellular components. The collagen is oriented parallel to the lines of stress, and tensile strength is increased. When these tissues are lengthened, the muscles are subjected to prolonged positioning in this new lengthened state, and the number of sarcomeres increases (McClure, et al., 1994). With this in mind, it appears that the primary rationale for using splints is to apply relatively long periods of tensile stress to shortened connective tissues, which will cause tissue lengthening through the biologic remodeling process (McClure, et al., 1994).

Now you are armed with a basic understanding of why tissue shortens, what causes it to relengthen, and a scientifically sound rationale for splint use. The one challenge remaining is to determine how long the splint should be worn each day and at what time intervals. It appears as though the splint wearing schedule can be either continuous (i.e., 8 consecutive hours each day), or cyclical (i.e. 2 hours on/2 hours off for a total of 8 hours each day) and still result in tissue lengthening. Studies show that controlled tensile stress applied either cyclically or statically leads to remodeling of periarticular tissue.

To make changes in range of motion, it is not important whether the splint is worn continuously or cyclically, but instead how long the joint is stressed at its end range. You can provide a joint with a low-load prolonged stress (LLPS) such as splinting, or with a high-load brief stress (HLBS) such as manual range of motion or joint manipulation. There have been many studies done comparing LLPS to HLBS, and the results consistently demonstrate that more significant changes in range are made with LLPS (McClure and Flowers, 1992). The definition of prolonged is different for each patient. The goal is to have the splint worn as many hours each day as it takes to increase range of motion without causing any detrimental effects such as pain or inflammation. The total amount of time the joint is held at or near its end range is called Total End Range Time (TERT), a term introduced by Flowers and Michlovitz (1988). To determine the TERT, multiply the *frequency* the splint is worn by the *duration* it is worn. For example, if a patient is wearing a splint four times per day, for 30 minutes each session, that equals a total of 120 minutes of TERT. In addition to the TERT, you must also consider the *intensity,* which is determined by the force or the angle of the splint.

These three factors—frequency, duration, and intensity—all play a role in the prescribed wearing schedule. So whether you select a continuous or cyclical wearing schedule, the key factor in influencing a change in the range of motion is the TERT. If you fear the patient will have a low tolerance to splint wear, start with a TERT of 1 hour per day (in any frequency). If there is no pain or skin integrity problems, but 1 hour of TERT is not making any change in the range of motion, increase the TERT. It is important to monitor the patient two to three times per week until a therapeutic amount of TERT is determined. You will know when it is therapeutic because improvements in range of motion will be evident, but the patient will not have pain or inflammation. Some recalcitrant contractures may require up to 16 hours of TERT each day (McClure and Flowers, 1992). Once the maximum TERT is achieved, you still have the ability to increase the intensity by changing the splint angle if continued range of motion is still the goal. An insufficient dose of stress will have no therapeutic effect on the child, and an excessive dose of stress will produce complications such as pain and inflammation. Patients with acute inflammation are not appropriate for end range splinting because prolonged end range stress would risk increasing the inflammatory response. Overall, it is believed that splinting using LLPS should be used when the limited range is due to structural changes in periarticular tissues and should not be used when the limited range is due to nonstructural changes such as pain and "guarding" (McClure and Flowers, 1992).

There are two primary reasons to discontinue splinting. These are 1) if the range of motion goals has been achieved and 2) if no increase in the range of motion has been achieved even when the splint was worn with maximum TERT and intensity for a prolonged period of time.

When establishing a wearing schedule for your patient, keep these principles in mind:
- Keep the purpose/goal of the splint in the forefront of your mind.
- Joints with a hard end feel (a sudden stop when attempting to move the extremity within a normal range) require more hours (TERT) than joints with a springy end feel.
- Limit initial use until skin tolerance is established and then build up the TERT to a therapeutic point. During this "build up phase," monitor the patient two to three times per week.
- LLPS produces better range of motion results than HLBS.
- LLPS should be used when the limited range is due to structural changes and not when due to nonstructural changes.
- Write down the wearing schedule for the caregiver.
- Make sure the wearing schedule is compatible and consistent with the child's normal routine.
- Periodic splint removal is necessary for skin inspection, exercise, and hygiene.

## Safety

The use of splints in pediatrics is an effective method for improving patient's function or positioning, decreasing hygiene problems, and decreasing self-injurious behavior. As with splinting adults, certain precautions should be observed to ensure the well-being of your patient. We all need to practice good judgment and concern about safety, particularly when splinting infants and small children who may not be able to tell you if they are uncomfortable or in pain, and who may not have the cognitive skills to prevent themselves from self-injury with the splint in place. The following are several safety tips that you should keep in mind when fabricating splints in a pediatric setting.

### Heat Pans and Warm Thermoplastics

Always remember, thermoplastic splinting materials were designed to be used at a particular temperature. Make sure that you are using the temperature recommended by the manufacturer when heating thermoplastics in a pan of water. Most materials heat between 150° and 170°. This is approximately the "warm/simmer" setting on an electric skillet, which many therapists use to heat their materials. Setting the dial on an electric skillet to 350° will not make your water heat any faster. The water has to heat to 170° before it can get to 350°. Heating your water by cranking it up to 300° or 350° does two things. It makes your material too hot, posing the risk of scorching your patient, and it affects the properties of your thermoplastic material. In other words, your favorite elastic performs perfectly at its recommended temperature, but get it too hot and it starts to lose its level of conformability or resistance to stretch. For these same reasons we don't recommend heating your material in a microwave oven or a pan of water on the stove. When you heat your material that way, you have little control over the temperature it is reaching or whether it is heating evenly.

Before placing the heated piece of thermoplastic material onto a child's sensitive skin, dry off the excess water and allow it to cool slightly. Let the child blow on it or touch it to decrease the level of apprehension about being splinted. If you are using a perforated material you *must* dry it on a counter with a cloth or paper towel to remove as much excess water from the holes as possible. Water trapped in the perforations may burn your patient. If you still have concerns about using a heated thermoplastic on a patient, try the following. Pre-form the splint and have it almost completely shaped before you place it on the child's hand. Wet the child's hand and arm with a washcloth dipped in cold water just prior to placing the warm material on the skin. Some therapists like to splint directly over a stockinette to diffuse the heat transferred from the thermoplastic material to the child's skin. We have found, however, that this can result in wrinkles or uneven textures in the interior of the splint. This happens because the stockinette has a tendency to fold or bunch when the thermoplastic is applied. This can cause discomfort for the child as he wears the splint and is a potential risk for pressure areas. Use caution if you use this technique. You can avoid the use of thermoplastics altogether and opt for a splint made of neoprene, orthopedic felt, or for very small infants, cloth tape.

## Avoid Choking

Children love to bring things to their mouths. For this reason you need to pay close attention to your splint and all its parts, straps included. Avoid small objects on a splint whenever possible, especially for an infant or preschool child or with children who have a history of putting objects in their mouths. If you must make a dynamic splint for a young child (which we usually don't recommend due to increased risk of injury and the fact that most young children are not capable of following the treatment/exercise program that typically accompanies a dynamic splint), use low-profile outriggers, avoid metal parts such as springs and wires, and avoid detachable items such as rubberbands. Thera-Band® Tubing™ or narrow strips of Thera-Band can be tied onto the splint in place of springs and rubberbands. (Be aware that these two products usually contain latex and some children, particularly those with spina bifida, may have an allergy to latex.) You can also use thin elastic or run your wire or nylon through thermoplastic tubes such as ThermoTubes™ or Aquatubes®. Always make sure your attachments are secure. When attaching one piece of a thermoplastic to another or attaching Velcro to thermoplastic, always use a heat gun to ensure that you have a strong bond. Any thermoplastic decorations on the splint should be appropriately attached in the same manner and rechecked frequently for safety.

## Toxicity

Pay attention to labels on the products you use. Select ones that are non-toxic whenever possible. When fabricating a neoprene splint, we prefer to use Scotch Permanent Adhesive Glue Stick when we can, but the adhesive isn't very tacky when wet, and it takes several hours to dry. Most neoprene glues claim to be non-toxic when they have dried. Manufacturers usually recommend that you apply the adhesive in a well-ventilated area because of the fumes. If you are going to decorate your neoprene splint with fabric paints, make sure that they, too, are non-toxic. (Fabric paint doesn't stick very well to thermoplastic splints. Therefore your patient could easily pick it off and possibly ingest it.) If you draw on or color a thermoplastic splint with permanent markers, use non-toxic ones. Most non-toxic markers are not permanent. However, Sammons Preston sells some splint markers that are non-toxic, permanent, and reasonably priced.

## General Safety Precautions

There are several common sense suggestions you should follow when splinting children. Round the edges of your thermoplastic splints so your patients will not scratch or poke themselves if they bring the splint to their face. When using a perforated material, smooth the edges so that the children do not scratch themselves with the perforations. You can do this by heating the cut edges of the splint and rubbing them firmly against a flat surface such as a table or counter. You also can apply a protective strip across the perforated edges such as Aquaplast Ultra Thin Edging Material. We recommend applying these easy-to-use strips with a heat gun, which results in a quick, durable bond.

Monitor the fit of your patient's splint regularly. Children, unlike adults, are constantly growing. It is likely they could outgrow their splint before they wear it out. A tight splint could impair your patient's circulation and cause pressure sores. Pay close attention to neoprene splints. Openings for the thumb or finger can become tight and result in the tip of the finger becoming cold or bluish in color. Usually this situation can be remedied by making a few cuts into the hole and opening it up slightly. If your patient's splint requires more than a few snips, it may have to be refabricated. You may be able to get a little more life out of your thermoplastic splint, depending upon where it is tight and what type of material it was made from. Cautiously reheating and refabricating small areas may enable you to open up thumb holes or forearm troughs on some splints.

Finally, pay close attention to your clinic surroundings. We know this can be hard to do when you're trying to fabricate a splint on a fidgety 2-year-old child with hemiplegia, but it is critical. Even if your patients are angelic and well-behaved, they may have siblings that find the clinic setting an interesting place to explore. Keep electric cords from your heating pan, heat gun, and iron out of reach. Don't let them dangle where a child could reach them and possibly pull a hot iron or a pan of hot water off the counter. Put away your scissors and utility knives. Keep all small objects out of reach. Read and follow the manufacturer's directions whenever possible.

In review, here are some suggestions for safety:
- Keep electric skillet set between 150° and 170°.
- Dry perforated materials well to remove water trapped in perforations.
- Avoid small objects on a splint.
- If you must make a dynamic splint, avoid high-profile outriggers, metal parts, and detachable items. Instead substitute Thera-Band Tubing, Thera-Band, or elastic.
- Make sure all attachments are securely bonded.
- Select non-toxic products whenever possible.
- Round all edges.
- Smooth or cover perforations that have been cut.
- Regularly monitor splints for fit on a growing child.
- Keep cords, sharp objects, and small items out of reach of children.
- Read and follow manufacturer's directions whenever possible.

## Stocking and Maintaining Your Clinic

In this time of shrinking budgets and limited resources, it is not always possible to surround yourself with all the supplies and equipment you desire. Being able to provide your clients with the ideal splint, while still being cost effective, can be a challenge. Therapists tend to develop personal preferences for particular thermoplastic materials. What works well for one therapist may be awkward and frustrating for another. Because of this inconsistency with preferences, it is best to experiment with as many different products as possible before committing to a large purchase. Attend splinting courses that include lab experiences and invite your local product representatives to your facility for material demonstrations and product inservices. These representatives are an excellent resource to learn about material properties and recommended uses.

Once you become more familiar with the materials and products available, it is time to stock your clinic. It would be ideal to have one of each type of thermoplastic: elastic-like, plastic-like, rubber-like, and plastic-rubber-like. If you splint newborns or children with progressive neuromuscular weakness or atrophy conditions, adding thin (1/16-inch or 1/12-inch) materials to your list is critical to keep your finished product lightweight. If you splint children with severely involved extremities where hygiene is frequently a problem, adding perforated materials to your supply would be a benefit. If purchasing materials in each of the four thermoplastic categories is not financially feasible, you may opt for only two materials: 1) elastic-like, which is very cost-effective because its excellent memory allows the same splint to be refabricated and reused several times, and 2) plastic-rubber-like, which is user friendly and considered the ideal "middle of the road" choice. It will provide you with a little of everything including a moderate level of control, a moderate degree of conformability/drapability, and a moderate degree of strength.

In addition to thermoplastic materials, neoprene is practically mandatory in pediatric clinics. If you have not yet had the opportunity to work with neoprene materials, be aware that they are available in a variety of thicknesses, colors, and material backings. To see what is available, contact a supplier and request sample swatches. Consider the needs of your clinic when determining what thicknesses and backings you will buy. The thinner materials will allow increased ease of movement and better conformability to the palm but will not provide as much aggressive alignment, support, or positioning. Conversely, the thicker neoprene materials will provide better alignment, support, and positioning but will inhibit movement, have less conformability to the palm, and may interfere with grasp and retention of small objects in the palm. When selecting a neoprene backing, consider its comfort against the child's skin, which backings will absorb perspiration, and which ones may create more of a perspiration problem.

In addition to these primary fabrication materials, other materials and supplies we have found to be useful in pediatric splinting are as follows:

- Adapt-It Thermoplastic Pellets
- Elastomer
- Elastomer Adhesive
- X-Lite (Hexcelite)
- Aquaplast Ultra Thin Edging Material
- clipboard (to serve as a hard surface to trace patient's hand for pattern making when a tabletop, wheelchair tray, or other surface is unavailable)
- loop Velcro (variety of colors)
- Self-adhesive hook Velcro

- Velfoam®, Beta Pile or similar strapping material
- Poly-Lock or Dual Lock
- Rubatex, neoprene glue/cement or Scotch™ Permanent Glue Stick
- large electric skillet (with pan liner)
- silent heat gun with nozzle
- utility knife
- non-toxic, colored permanent markers
- shoelaces, shoelace keepers, and diaper clips
- small finger rivets
- therapy putty (medium firmness)
- spatula
- baster
- liquid soap
- neoprene tape (Melco tape)
- clothing iron
- fabric paints
- Quik-Freeze or Cold Spray
- curved splinting scissors
- regular scissors
- scissors for self-adhesive Velcro
- revolving hole punch
- grease pencil (light color)
- industrial paper towels
- sewing thread and needle
- elastic bandage wrap, Coban
- Thera-Band

## Maintaining Your Clinic

At the risk of sounding like your mother, we must state the obligatory "put your things away." This simple advice is probably the easiest offered but most often ignored advice around (Figure 3.13). In terms of cost-effectiveness, those materials and tools that are put away will be available for use later, and those materials and tools that are not put away often grow feet and walk away on their own accord.

See if this sounds familiar: You need to make a splint. You open the splinting cupboard to select a material and as you gaze into the cupboard, you see an array of splinting materials. There's the white stuff that has a shiny gloss to it, then there's the white stuff with the not-so-shiny coating, and then there's the perforated white stuff, all of which are unidentifiable. Hmmmm . . . which white stuff to pick? If you knew what you were looking at, you might be able to make an appropriate choice.

Unfortunately, this is an all too common scenario. Busy therapists do not always have the luxury of labeling thermoplastic materials each and every time they return one to the splinting cupboard. However, we could probably all find 15 minutes one time per year to sit down and label a sheet of peel-off stickers. These could then be hung inside the cupboard door. This way, every time you cut a piece of material and return the remainder to the cupboard you only have to find 2 additional seconds to peel off a sticker with the word *Orfit, Orthoplast* etc., written on it and quickly adhere it to the piece you are

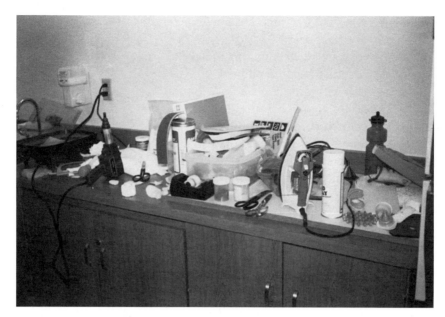

Figure **3.13** Don't let this happen to you! Unsafe and inefficient workspace interferes with successful splinting

returning to the cupboard. If you want, you could also code your stickers with different colors representing different thermoplastic categories (i.e., green = elastics; red = plastics; yellow = rubbers; blue = plastic-rubbers). If this system is not feasible at your clinic, you could at least label bins with material names so that each therapist is more likely to return unused portions and scraps to the correct bin.

Another tip is to keep a running list of desired materials posted in your splinting area with a pen or pencil attached to a string. Each time you think of a material or tool that would make your splinting easier or more successful, you can add it to the list. In addition, when you notice the clinic is running low on a particular item, you are more likely to remember to reorder it if you immediately write it on the materials list. This way whenever it is time to order materials you do not have to take an hour out of your busy schedule to sort through the materials cupboard and peruse the manufacturers' catalogs; your list is already done.

You also should try to keep one pair of scissors designated as the self-adhesive Velcro scissors. When scissors cut through the adhesive backing, glue builds up on their blades. This can be frustrating when you try to cut regular Velcro, Velfoam, or neoprene with these same scissors. When glue does accumulate on your scissors blades, rubbing alcohol, Goo Gone, or nail polish remover can be used to dissolve the glue. Remember that all of these products are toxic and should be used with caution, especially if your client is present during cleaning. When using a neoprene glue such as Rubatex or Seal Cement, it is important to remember to thoroughly clean the mouth of the jar, the lid, and the brush prior to replacing the lid or your can of adhesive will not reopen. Using these cement glues is not a cost-effective choice if the can becomes "single use" because it cannot be reopened.

Once these tips for maintaining your clinic become habit, you will find that your splinting becomes faster and more successful as a result of having easy access to all of the necessary materials and tools.

# Splint Patterns and Fabrication Directions

Chapter **4**

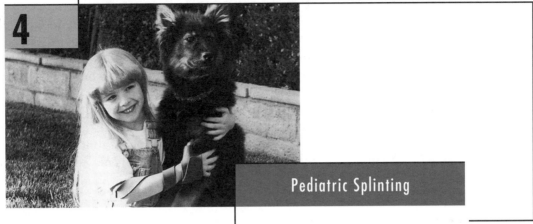

Pediatric Splinting

This chapter is devoted to fabrication of pediatric splints. You will find fabrication instructions for 28 splints, accompanied by a pattern when appropriate. Whenever possible, the splint pattern should be customized by tracing your patient's extremity and marking appropriate anatomical landmarks as suggested in the fabrication instructions. There are a few patterns that are difficult to draw directly from a tracing of the patient's extremity. In these cases the pattern size must be estimated and then reduced or enlarged as needed. We recommend that you read through the fabrication instructions at least once before attempting to fabricate the splint. You will be most successful if you read the instructions and have all your supplies prepared *before* beginning fabrication. Remember to be creative. Experiment with these patterns and modify them as appropriate to meet each client's needs.

## Sof-Splint

### Purpose

This splint inhibits thumb adduction without blocking functional thumb opposition.

### Recommended Patient

This splint design is intended for use with the patient who has mildly to moderately increased muscle tone or other conditions resulting in a mildly adducted thumb. It may be fabricated for patients with cerebral palsy, a brachial plexus injury, or head trauma. This splint also can be used with some cases of arthrogryposis when the "thumb in palm" is secondary to muscular or soft tissue causes but not when it is secondary to bony deformities or contractures. The design allows movement at the CMC joint and therefore is an excellent functional splint. It is not recommended for patients with severely increased muscle tone or contractures because there is not enough force provided by the thumb loop to inhibit thumb adduction. It is not a static splint but rather semi-dynamic in design.

### Supplies and Materials

Neo-Plush and regular hook Velcro are the best materials for this splint. Neoprene, with a pile or terry cloth backing, can be used in place of Neo-plush. When using a material like Neo-Plush, you can attach the hook Velcro anywhere along the Neo-Plush surface because Neo-Plush provides a "built in" mate for hook Velcro. This enables you to make minor positional changes and control tension without having to constantly resew Velcro onto the strap to modify your splint.

You will need additional materials to attach the Velcro to the Neo-Plush or neoprene. Depending on your preference, select either iron-on Velcro (0143) or sewing thread and a needle. If the neoprene you select does not have pile backing, you also will need regular loop Velcro to mate with the hook Velcro.

### Instructions for Splint or Pattern Making

This simple splint consists of two neoprene straps, one for the wrist and one for the thumb. First, measure the circumference of your client's wrist and cut a neoprene strap this length plus one additional inch to allow overlap for the Velcro closure attachment. The width of this wrist strap can vary according to how much stability you need; 1/2-inch to 3/4-inch usually is adequate. Attach one piece of hook Velcro as a closure for the wrist strap. For the thumb strap, measure the distance from the dorsum of the wrist, through the web space, over the thenar eminence, and then back to the dorsum of the wrist and cut a second neoprene strap this exact length. Attach hook Velcro to the dorsum of the wrist strap upon which you anchor both ends of the thumb loop (see Figure 4.3 on page 82).

There are several variations of this splint. Using the wrist strap as an anchor, you can attach one end of the thumb strap to the dorsum of the wrist as in the previous instructions but use a figure-eight wrap around the base of the thumb. Attach the other end to the volar surface of the wrist band (Figure 4.1). This figure-eight wrap provides additional support to the dorsal side of the thumb MP joint and prevents hyperextension at this joint, which is a potential problem with the original design (Figure 4.2).

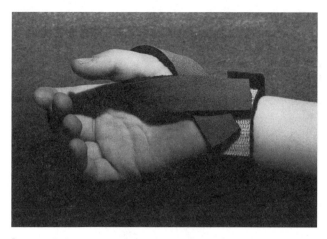

Figure **4.1** A modified figure-eight wrap provides support across the dorsal side of the thumb MP joint

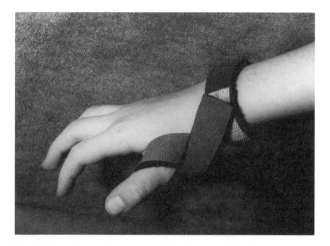

Figure **4.2** A dorsal view of the modified figure-eight wrap

The advantage of using two separate straps is that the therapist can easily grade the amount of tension or torque created to radially abduct the thumb while still maintaining it in proper alignment. Another option to grade the amount of support provided is to vary the thickness of the neoprene. Use thinner material for the mildly affected thumb and thicker material for the more moderately affected thumb.

## REFERENCES

Reymann, J. (1985). The Sof-splint. *Developmental Disabilities Special Interest Section Newsletter, 8*(2), 1–2.

A similar pre-fabricated splint can be purchased commercially from the Joe Cool Company™. This company has neoprene thumb splints available in preemie to adult sizes in a variety of fun, bright colors. The price is $11–$15, which includes shipping and handling.

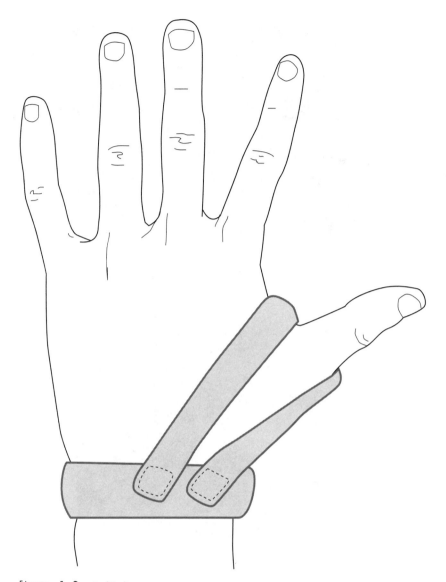

Figure **4.3**  Sof-Splint

Copyright © 1998 by Therapy Skill Builders, a division of The Psychological Corporation/All rights reserved/
Laura Hogan and Tracey Uditsky, Pediatric Splinting/ISBN 0761615148/1-800-228-0752/This page is reproducible.

# Standard Neoprene Thumb-Abduction Splint

## Purpose

Use this splint to position the thumb in a more abducted and extended position to enable the child to have better opposition for prehension. It can also be used to increase range of motion. Because the neoprene is a soft material, it permits some active range of motion during function.

## Recommended Patient

There are a wide variety of patients for whom this splint may be beneficial. This splint works very well for patients with mild interference from abnormal muscle tone at the thumb. It covers a relatively small amount of the hand, enabling the child to grasp, as well as receive some sensory input into the palm. You also can use this splint on children with moderate to severe spasticity. Because of the straight seam at the web space, it might be easier to get this splint on a spastic hand than some of the other neoprene splints with contour at the web space. However, if you choose this splint for a child with a significant thumb-in-palm position, it may increase range but not provide adequate positioning for function.

## Supplies and Materials

You will need a piece of neoprene 4 to 6 inches in length and 2 to 4 inches wide. The thickness and texture will vary based on the desired results and individual characteristics of your patient. For small children or children with mild spasticity, a 1/8-inch thickness usually is sufficient. For older, elementary school children or children with moderate spasticity, 1/4-inch works well. If you fabricate this splint for a child with moderate to severe spasticity in the thumb adductors, we recommend a thicker neoprene such as 3/8-inch. You also will need needle and thread, or a neoprene adhesive and 3 to 5 inches of Melco tape (also known as neoprene tape). Select some type of fastener such as Velcro hook and loop. One fastener or strap usually is sufficient for this splint.

## Instructions for Splint or Pattern Making

This splint is quick and simple to make. The pattern provided can be enlarged or reduced as needed to fit your patient's hand. We keep several pattern sizes on hand to try on our patients. To make your own pattern, follow the steps listed here.

Place the child's hand on a piece of paper. Extend the thumb and open up the web space as much as possible. Trace the hand. (If you can't get the thumb out adequately, simulate extension when you trace the hand.) Mark the following anatomical landmarks: the MP of the index finger, the IP of the thumb on both its ulnar and radial sides, and the MP of the thumb. To make the pattern, mark points A, B, C, and D as shown in Figure 4.6 on page 85. Make point A on the hand just proximal to the head of the metacarpal of the index finger. Make points B, C, and D as shown approximately 1/4-inch to 3/8-inch from the hand to ensure that the thumb hole won't be too tight.

Draw a line from point A to point B and then from point C to point D. These two lines will be your seams when fabricating the splint. Draw a line across the thumb between points B and C. This line represents the thumb opening. (When the splint is on the child,

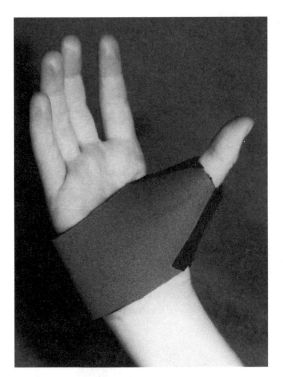

Figure **4.4** Volar view of splint, thumb portion ends proximal to the IP crease to allow IP flexion

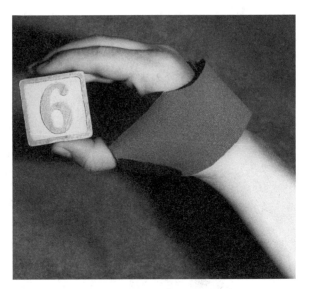

Figure **4.5** Laterial view demonstrating improved alignment for functional use of the hand

you will want the fabric to clear the IP crease so the child can flex freely at that joint for grasping.) The main portion of your pattern is now complete. Simply draw a line from point A, just proximal to the knuckles, to the ulnar side of the child's hand. Round the edges as shown and draw another line to point D.

You will cut this pattern from neoprene twice. It is used for both the palmar and dorsal pieces of the splint. Place the pattern on the outside (or lycra side) of the neoprene and trace the dorsal piece. Flip the pattern over and trace the palmar piece. Connect the two seams in the manner you prefer. You may sew them by hand or machine or iron on the Melco (neoprene) tape. Using the tape with this splint design is particularly easy because both seams are straight (see How To Work With Neoprene in Chapter 3 for information on how to use Melco tape). Apply a fastener of your choice. The completed splint is shown in Figures 4.4 and 4.5.

### REFERENCES

Original design for the neoprene thumb-abduction splint courtesy of Deborah Earich, O.T.R.; Michele S. Jones, P.T., and Wayne Wilkerson, C.P.

The Joe Cool Company sells a pre-fabricated splint similar to this one called the Hand Glove. It comes in a wide selection of colors. Prices are from $15 to $20 (plus shipping and handling) and sizes range from preemie to adult.

The Benik Corporation will custom make a variety of neoprene splints based on dimensions and specifications that you provide. Splints can be fabricated similar to this design as well as numerous others. Prices range from $9 to $26 (plus shipping and handling). Benik also sells neoprene in a variety of fun colors by the square foot, as well as Melco tape (neoprene tape) by the inch.

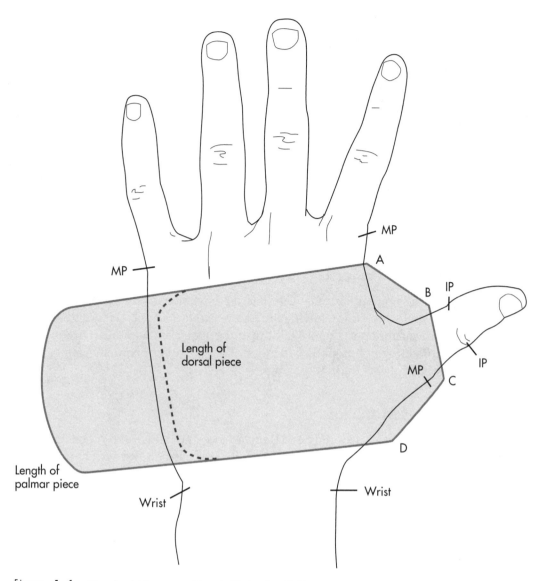

Figure **4.6**   Standard Neoprene Thumb-Abduction Splint

Copyright © 1998 by Therapy Skill Builders, a division of The Psychological Corporation/All rights reserved/
Laura Hogan and Tracey Uditsky, Pediatric Splinting/ISBN 0761615148/1-800-228-0752/This page is reproducible.

## Modified Neoprene Thumb-Abduction Splint with Wrist Component

### Purpose

Use this splint to open up the web space and position the thumb into a more abducted and extended position to enable the child to have better use of the hand. You also can use it to increase range of motion.

This splint aligns the fingers for pinch, but the bulk of material in the palm of the hand may interfere somewhat with palmar grasping. Because of the length of this splint, it provides some support at the wrist. It covers substantial surface area of the palm and wrist and serves as an excellent "glove" under which the therapist may place a variety of inserts such as a web spacer, ulnar gutter, or palmar support. Thermoplastic stays also can be attached to the outside of the splint if desired. It is a soft splint that permits some active range of motion.

### Recommended Patient

Because of the contour at both the web space and the lateral side of the thumb, this splint can be used with children with a moderate amount of spasticity in the hand. It provides more support at the MP joint than the standard neoprene thumb-abduction splint, but still does not immobilize the joint. Like the other neoprene splints, this splint is comfortable for most children to wear.

### Supplies and Materials

You will need a piece of neoprene 4 to 9 inches in length and 4 to 6 inches wide. The thickness and texture of the neoprene will vary based on the desired results and individual characteristics of your patient. Generally 1/4-inch works well. If you fabricate this splint for a child with moderate to severe spasticity you may want to use a thicker neoprene. You also will need thread and needle, or a neoprene adhesive and 5 to 8 inches of Melco tape (neoprene tape). Select some type of fastener such as Velcro hook and loop. Two fasteners or straps usually are sufficient for this splint. If inserts and stays are to be used they can be fabricated out of elastomer putty, Adapt-it Thermoplastic Pellets, or a variety of thermoplastic materials.

### Instructions for Splint or Pattern Making

Place the child's hand on a piece of paper. Extend the thumb and open up the web space as much as possible. Trace the hand. (If you can't get the thumb out adequately, simulate extension when you trace the hand.) Mark the following anatomical landmarks: the MP joint of the index and the little fingers, the IP of the thumb on both its ulnar and radial sides, and both sides of the wrist. To make the pattern, mark points A through F as shown in Figure 4.9 on page 89. Points D and E are 1 to 2 inches proximal to the carpal metacarpal joints (wrist joint). Make points A, B, C, and D as shown approximately 1/8-inch to 3/8-inch from the hand to ensure that the splint is not too tight. Draw one line from point A to point B and one line from point C to point D. These two lines represent your seams. Follow the contours of the child's hand, but make the line smooth or you will have a difficult time joining the two pieces of neoprene at that seam. Draw a line across the thumb between points B and C. This line represents the thumb opening.

(When the splint is on the child you will want the fabric to clear the IP crease so the child can flex freely at that joint for grasping.) Now draw a line from point A to point F just proximal to the knuckles. Draw a line from point D to point E, and point E to point F as shown.

**Important Tip:** The distance from the outline of the child's hand to the marks for the pattern will vary depending upon the thickness of the child's hand and the thickness of the neoprene. For this splint, if you intend to use inserts you must also allow some extra room in the pattern. Planning for more room at the web space is critical, particularly when using a thick insert such as elastomer putty or Adapt-It Thermoplastic Pellets. Neoprene 1/4-inch thick combined with an insert may necessitate that you draw your pattern lines as much as 1/2-inch from the anatomical landmarks. Err on the side of too large when making a pattern; the neoprene can always be trimmed.

Cut this pattern from neoprene twice. Like the other neoprene splints, it is used for both the palmar and dorsal pieces of the splint. Cut the palmar piece longer than the dorsal piece so you have about 1 inch overlapped, providing you with adequate space for straps.

Connect the two seams in the manner you prefer. You may sew them by hand or by machine. The seams can be made using the Melco (neoprene) tape, but because of the curves in both seams, this can be awkward and time consuming if you are unfamiliar with the technique. Apply fasteners of your choice. We recommend one at the proximal and one at the distal edge of the splint. You may want to add a third strap in between if your patient is large. Remember, when attaching straps you want to pull the neoprene from the dorsal piece to the palmar piece so you are pulling the thumb into extension (see How To Work with Neoprene in Chapter 3). The completed splint is shown in Figures 4.7 and 4.8.

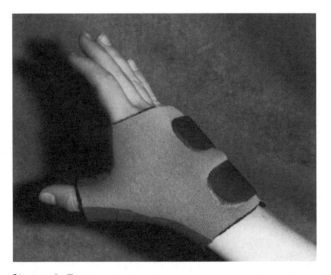

Figure **4.7** Lateral view showing contour at the web space

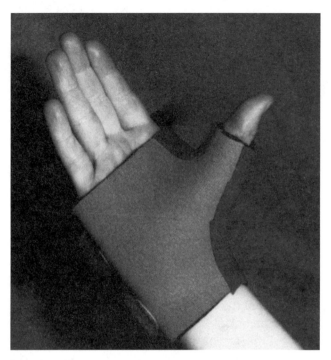

Figure **4.8** Volar view. This splint covers substantial surface area of the palm and wrist and serves as an excellent "glove" under which you can place a variety of inserts

## REFERENCES

The authors designed this splint.

The Benik Corporation will make a variety of neoprene splints based on dimensions and specifications that you provide. They can be fabricated similar to this design as well as numerous others. Prices range from $9 to $26 (plus shipping and handling). Benik will add stays and pockets if requested. The company also sells neoprene in a variety of fun colors by the square foot, as well as Melco tape (neoprene tape) by the inch.

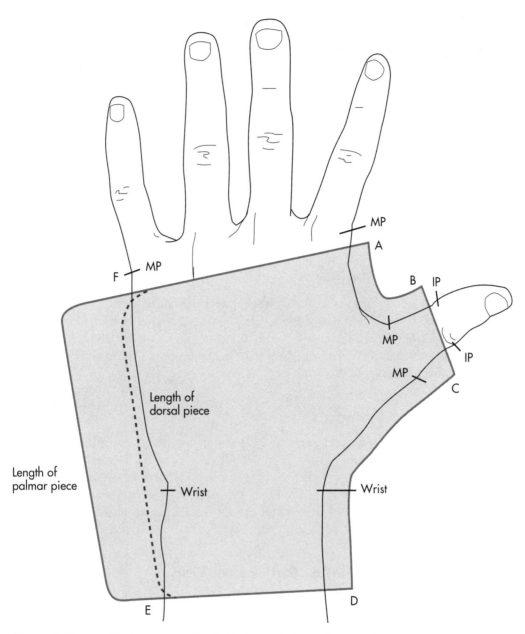

Figure **4.9** Modified Neoprene Thumb-Abduction Splint with Wrist Component

Copyright © 1998 by Therapy Skill Builders, a division of The Psychological Corporation/All rights reserved/
Laura Hogan and Tracey Uditsky, Pediatric Splinting/ISBN 0761615148/1-800-228-0752/This page is reproducible.

## Modified Neoprene Thumb-Abduction Splint
### Purpose

This splint is used to open up the web space and position the thumb into a more abducted and extended position to enable the child to have better use of the hand.

This is the same pattern as the modified neoprene thumb-abduction splint with wrist component except it is shorter. It aligns the fingers for pinch, but the bulk of material in the palm of the hand may interfere somewhat with palmar grasping. This splint ends at the wrist, enabling the child to flex and extend actively at the wrist. It covers substantial surface area at the palm and serves as an excellent "glove" under which the therapist may choose to place a variety of inserts such as a web spacer or palmar support. It is a soft splint that permits some active range of motion. This splint is also the one we prefer to use for the base of the neoprene thumb-abduction supination splint (TASS).

### Recommended Patient

Because of the contour at both the web space and the lateral side of the thumb, this splint can be used with children with a moderate amount of spasticity in the hand. It provides more support at the MP joint than the standard neoprene thumb-abduction splint but still does not immobilize the joints. Like the other neoprene splints, this splint is comfortable for most children to wear.

### Supplies and Materials

You will need a piece of neoprene 3 to 5 inches in length and 4 to 6 inches wide. The thickness and texture of the neoprene will vary based on the desired results and individual characteristics of your patient; generally 1/4-inch works well. If you fabricate this splint for a child with moderate to severe spasticity you may want to use a thicker neoprene. You will also need thread and needle or a neoprene adhesive and 4 to 6 inches of Melco tape (neoprene tape). Select some type of fastener such as Velcro hook and loop.

### Instructions for Splint or Pattern Making

Place the child's hand on a piece of paper. Extend the thumb and open up the web space as much as possible. Trace the hand. (If you can't get the thumb out adequately, simulate extension when you trace the hand.) Mark the following anatomical landmarks: the MP joint of the index and the little fingers, the IP of the thumb on both its ulnar and radial sides, and both sides of the wrist. To make the pattern, mark A through F as shown in Figure 4.11 on page 92. Points D and E are just distal to the carpal metacarpal joints (wrist joint). Make points A, B, C, and D as shown approximately 1/8-inch to 1/4-inch from the hand to ensure that the splint is not too tight. Draw one line from point A to point B; draw another from point C to point D. These two lines represent your seams. Follow the contour of the outline of the child's hand, but make the line smooth or you will have a difficult time joining the two pieces of neoprene at that seam. Draw a line across the thumb between points B and C. This line represents the thumb opening. (When the splint is on the child you will want the fabric to clear the IP crease so the child can flex freely at that joint for grasping.) Now draw a line from point A to point F just proximal to the knuckles. Draw a line from point D to point E and point E to point F as shown.

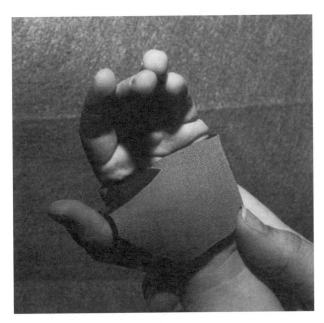

Figure **4.10**   Volar view of the modified neoprene thumb-abduction splint, which can be used as the base of the TASS

**Important Tip:** The distance from the outline of the child's hand to the marks for the pattern will vary depending upon the thickness of the child's hand and the thickness of the neoprene. For this splint, if you intend to use inserts you must also allow some extra room in the pattern. Planning for more room at the web space is critical, particularly when using a thick insert such as elastomer putty or Adapt-It Thermoplastic Pellets. Neoprene 1/4-inch thick combined with an insert may necessitate that you draw your pattern lines as much as 1/2-inch from the anatomical landmarks. Err on the side of too large when making a pattern, the neoprene can always be trimmed.

Cut this pattern from neoprene twice. Like the other neoprene splints, it is used for both the palmar and dorsal pieces of the splint. Cut the palmar piece longer than the dorsal piece so you have about 1 inch overlapped. This provides you with adequate space for straps.

Connect the two seams in the manner you prefer. You may sew them by hand or by machine. The seams can be made using the Melco (neoprene) tape, but because of the curves in both seams, this can be quite awkward and time-consuming if you are unfamiliar with this technique. Apply fasteners of your choice. We recommend one at the proximal edge and one at the distal edge of the splint. Remember, when attaching fasteners or straps you want the direction of pull to be from the dorsal piece to the palmar piece so you are pulling the thumb into extension (see How To Work with Neoprene in Chapter 3). The completed splint is shown in Figure 4.10.

### REFERENCES

The authors designed this splint.
The Benik Corporation will make a variety of neoprene splints, including one similar to this design. Prices range from $9 to $26 (plus shipping and handling). Benik will add stays and pockets if requested.

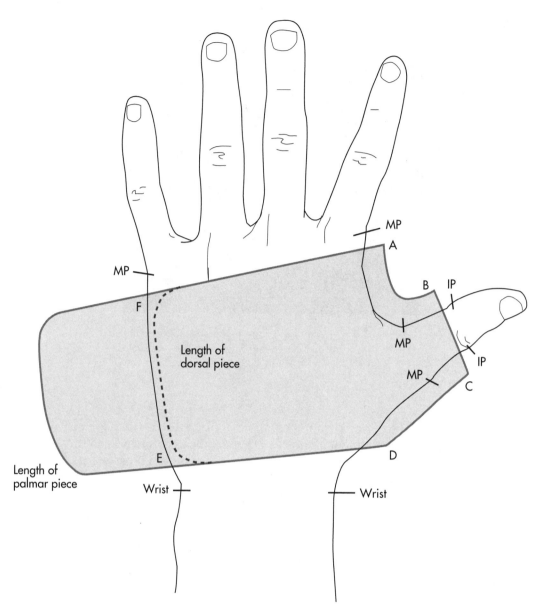

Figure **4.11** Modified Neoprene Thumb-Abduction Splint

Copyright © 1998 by Therapy Skill Builders, a division of The Psychological Corporation/All rights reserved/
Laura Hogan and Tracey Uditsky, Pediatric Splinting/ISBN 0761615148/1-800-228-0752/This page is reproducible.

# Thumb-Abduction Supination Splint (TASS)

## Purpose

This splint is used to open up the web space, position the thumb for improved opposition, and supinate the forearm for improved hand placement and function.

This splint uses the modified neoprene thumb-abduction splint or the standard neoprene thumb-abduction splint as its base. A neoprene strap is wrapped on the forearm to pull the arm into supination. For this reason, please refer to those patterns for your supplies list and directions. Only additional supplies and directions will be provided here.

## Recommended Patient

This is a useful splint for children with mild to moderate spasticity in the hand and arm. It is also recommended for children with brachial plexus injury. It provides improved positioning for function on children with potential for functional hand use. Although the supinator strap crosses the wrist at the dorsal surface, it usually does not have enough force to correct positioning at the wrist if the child has severe spasticity or flexion contractures at that joint.

## Supplies and Materials

You will need a 1- to 2-inch wide strip of neoprene 12 to 24 inches long, depending on the size of your patient. Additional Velcro hook and loop is needed to attach the strap at the hand and elbow.

## Instructions for Splint or Pattern Making

Fabricate your preferred neoprene thumb splint as the base according to the directions provided. Wrap the forearm strap once or twice around the forearm (we prefer two wraps for even more pull into supination). It crosses over the elbow and attaches to itself on the humerus. The easiest way to measure the length of neoprene needed for the strap is to use a cloth measuring tape and wrap it around the forearm and humerus in the same way you plan to wrap the strap. Once the forearm strap is cut, attach a 1-inch piece of Velcro loop to the underside of both ends of the strap. (If you are making this splint out of Neo-Plush or neoprene with a terry-cloth backing, you do not need to add the Velcro loop.) Attach a piece of Velcro hook to the dorsum of the thumb splint in a diagonal direction as indicated in Figure 4.12. Attach a second piece of hook on the outside of the strap where it overlaps onto itself proximal to the elbow.

To adjust the strap once the thumb portion is in place do the following. Place the distal end of the strap onto the thumb splint. Wrap the splint around the forearm once or twice, across the back of the elbow and around the humerus. As you wrap, pull the forearm into supination. Attach the splint to itself in a "cuff" fashion above the elbow (Figure 4.13). Now go back to the distal attachment and tighten or loosen the forearm strap and the amount of supination as needed.

Special Notes: There is another variation to this splint you might want to try. Instead of attaching the strap distally on the dorsum of the thumb splint, you can have a slightly longer strap that continues across the dorsum of the hand, across the web space, and into the palm. This type of strapping provides extra web opening if this is a major goal of your

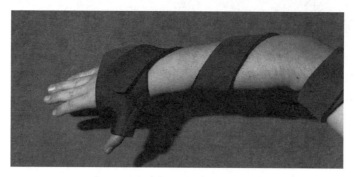

Figure **4.12**  Dorsal view of distal attachment of the forearm splint onto the dorsum of a modified neoprene thumb abduction splint

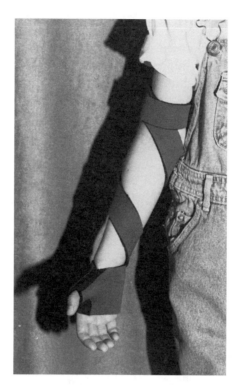

Figure **4.13**  Volar view demonstrating the forearm supination that can be obtained with the TASS. The end of the strap attaches to itself to form a "cuff" above the elbow

splint. However, it also adds quite a bit of bulk to the palm of the splint and can inhibit hand use for that reason. You might want to select this alternate strapping method on a child with limited functional hand use but who needs to gain some range of motion at the thumb and forearm. If needed, you can reverse the direction of pull of the strap and use it to gain pronation if your patient has a problem with excessive supination.

## REFERENCES

Original design for supination strap courtesy of Christine Alstadt Casey, OTR, Casey, C. A., & E. J. Kratz. (1988). Soft splinting with neoprene: the thumb abduction supinator splint. *American Journal of Occupational Therapy, 42*(6), 395–398.

Rehabilitation Division, Smith & Nephew, Inc. sells a pre-fabricated splint called the Rolyan® Tone And Positioning (TAP™) Splint. It is a two-piece design similar to the variation discussed previously in which the strap goes across the web space and attaches in the hand. This splint comes in pediatric sizes and sells for $35 to $40.

# Saddle Splint

## Purpose

This splint is used to open up the thumb web space and position the thumb in an abducted and opposed position.

## Recommended Patient

This splint works well for children who have mild to moderate muscle tone in the hand and show potential to use the hand functionally if they could align the thumb with the pads of the fingertips for grasping. This splint covers very little surface area of the hand. It allows good ventilation to the hand and leaves the palm relatively open for functional activities. Because the splint is small and does not disperse pressure across the hand, it will most likely be uncomfortable for children with severely spastic thumb flexors and adductors and is therefore not recommended for these children.

## Supplies and Materials

This is a small, easy-to-fabricate splint. Almost any scrap of thermoplastic material can be used; an elastic or rubber material works nicely. Use a 1/16-inch material for children who only require a little control and use up to 1/8-inch material for children who need more control. You will also need 12 to 16 inches of a soft, comfortable, non-stretchy strapping material like Velfoam, Velcro Dura-Loop, orthopedic felt, or Beta Pile in 3/4-inch width, and some Velcro hook and loop.

Important Note: Because there is not much surface area to the splint itself, there is potential for excessive pressure along the proximal and distal edges and on the lateral borders. When selecting your thermoplastic material, choose one on which you can easily finish the edges. If you use a perforated material, remember that the perforations, when cut, can create sharp edges.

## Instructions for Splint or Pattern Making

The design of the splint is in the form of a mask when flat and a saddle when completed, hence the name "saddle splint." Cut a paper towel in the shape of the pattern provided (see Figure 4.17 on page 98) and place it over the web space of your patient's thumb. The "sides of the saddle" rest on the thenar eminence and a small portion of the dorsal surface of the hand. At the web space, the saddle goes from the MP joint of the thumb to the distal palmar transverse crease by the index finger. (Because children's web spaces tend to be tight and immobile, spend a few minutes preparing the thumb before you begin splinting.) Once your splint pattern fits the web space, cut your thermoplastic material. You don't have to worry about the volar and dorsal sides of the splint at this time. They can be trimmed easily once you have shaped the web space portion of the splint.

When forming the splint, be sure to position the patient's thumb into opposition and abduction for function. Use your fingers to get a good curve in the web space (Figure 4.14). After the thumb portion is formed, mark and trim the material at the volar and dorsal sides. The volar side of the saddle generally does not extend farther than the thenar crease so it will not interfere with hand function when the thumb is abducted and opposed. The size and shape of the dorsal side of the saddle will not need much trimming or shaping. Its main purpose is to anchor the splint.

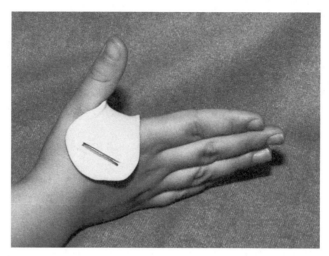

Figure **4.14** Dorsal lateral view demonstrating the thermoplastic material conformed to the web space

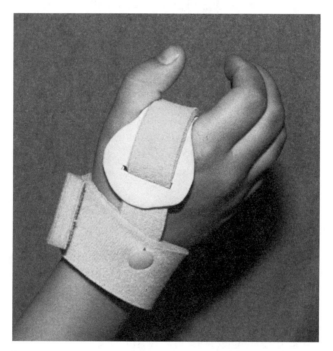

Figure **4.15** The strap for the web space is attached on the dorsal surface with a rivet. It goes up through the slot on the dorsal surface of the splint, over the web space, and down through the slot on the volar surface to help hold the splint in place

To fabricate the straps you first will need to make a wrist cuff with a Velcro closure. Then, using a rotary punch and a utility knife, make a 3/4-inch slot in each side of the saddle. Angle the slots so that the straps help anchor the splint on the hand as shown in the figures. Starting on the dorsal side, sew or otherwise permanently attach a 3/4-inch wide soft strap to the dorsal side of the wrist cuff (Figure 4.15). Run the strap through the splint from the dorsal slot, over the web space, and down through the slot on the volar side. Attach this strap with Velcro on the volar surface of the wrist cuff (Figure 4.16).

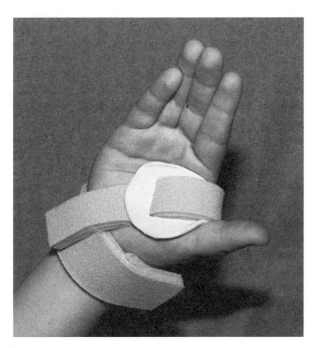

Figure **4.16** The strap for the web space attaches on the wrist cuff with a Velcro closure

There are lots of other ways you can attach straps to this splint. If you are making this splint for a very small child and there is not enough room for a 3/4-inch slot, you can create a smaller slot and trim your strap width accordingly. You also can make a small hole and run a shoelace through it and over the splint. You can rivet the straps to the splint if you prefer. Fasten one from the dorsal aspect of the saddle to the wrist cuff and another from the volar aspect of the saddle to the wrist cuff. If you use this method, the splint is attached permanently to the wrist cuff. Just make sure your direction of pull from the splint to the wrist cuff is correct and comfortable for the child. You don't have to make straps for this splint at all. You can use the basic design of the pattern and fabricate a thermoplastic insert that can be worn under a neoprene thumb-abductor splint (either custom or prefabricated) to provide extra support and control at the thumb web space. The neoprene will keep the insert in place. If you use the splint as an insert, pay even closer attention to creating smooth edges on the splint. You may need to apply moleskin or otherwise finish the edges.

**REFERENCES**
The authors designed this splint.

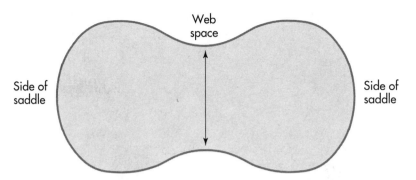

Figure **4.17** Saddle Splint

Copyright © 1998 by Therapy Skill Builders, a division of The Psychological Corporation/All rights reserved/
Laura Hogan and Tracey Uditsky, Pediatric Splinting/ISBN 0761615148/1-800-228-0752/This page is reproducible.

# Thumb Spica Splint

## Purpose

This splint is used to immobilize the thumb at the MP joint and properly align the thumb into a position of function. This splint usually is worn during the day during functional activities. It also may be used to decrease a flexion contracture at the thumb MP joint as well as provide a mild to moderate stretch to the soft tissues of the palm and support the arches.

## Recommended Patient

This splint works nicely for children who have too much spastic muscle tone to receive substantial benefit from the various types of neoprene thumb-adduction splints. It is also recommended for children with a hypermobile or unstable MP joint. Because it is made from a conforming thermoplastic material that covers the palm, you can stretch the fascia of the hand and build in appropriate arches if needed. Because it is a hard splint, it does not allow for active range of motion of the thumb MP or CMC joints. With the thumb positioned in slight abduction and opposition, weight bearing for extended periods of time may not be comfortable for the child.

## Supplies and Materials

Use a thin, elastic material for this splint; 1/12-inch micro-perforated soft Orfit works great. Because of the nature of the fabrication process, the material must self-bond at the lateral border of the thumb. One strap of Velcro loop is needed as is a small piece of self-adhesive Velcro hook.

## Instructions for Splint or Pattern Making

You do not need to fabricate a pattern for each child. Use the pattern provided and enlarge or reduce as needed. Have a few different sizes available to hold up to the back of your patient's hand. Precise sizing is not required, as excess material can be easily trimmed or rolled away. The only necessary measurement is from the lateral border of the MP joint of the index finger to about three-fourths the distance across the back of the hand. The pattern should be about that length from the cut at the web space (A) to the bottom (B) (see Figure 4.22 on page 102).

The most difficult part of making this splint is using your perceptual motor skills to place and form it on the child's hand. Position your patient's forearm into a neutral position (0° supination and pronation) with the thumb straight up and the fingers extended if possible. Place the warm material on the lateral side of the index finger just proximal to the distal palmar transverse crease (Figure 4.18).

Let the material "fall" backward into the web space and then pinch the two sides together as they wrap around the thumb as shown in Figure 4.19. This pinched edge eventually will be trimmed away. Now take the two flaps of the splint and wrap them around the palm and dorsum of the child's hand. The distal edge of the palmar portion of the splint should clear the distal palmar transverse crease.

**Important Note:** While forming this portion of the splint, have the child hold a small object. If this is not possible, be certain to position the thumb into opposition with the second and third finger to ensure that the child will have functional hand use while wearing the splint.

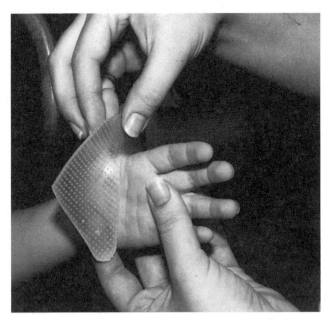

Figure **4.18**  With forearm in a neutral position, place material on lateral side of index finger just proximal to the distal palmar transverse crease

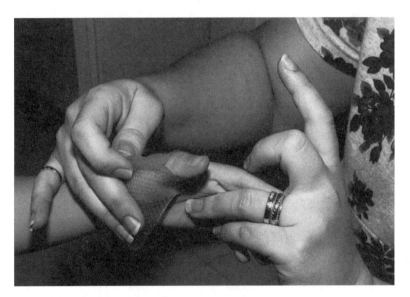

Figure **4.19**  Once material is positioned on the hand, form the web space portion and pinch the two sides together to circumferentially wrap the material around the thumb

As you continue to work with the palmar portion of the splint, you may form arches and get a good stretch into the fascia of the palm. To finish the splint, trim the excess at the radial border of the thumb. (Orfit will bond to itself and make a strong seam. You can reinforce it with Ultra Thin Edging if desired.) Roll back or trim the edges that interfere with function or that cause red marks. Attach one strap from the dorsal to the palmar piece at the ulnar side of the hand as shown in Figures 4.20 and 4.21.

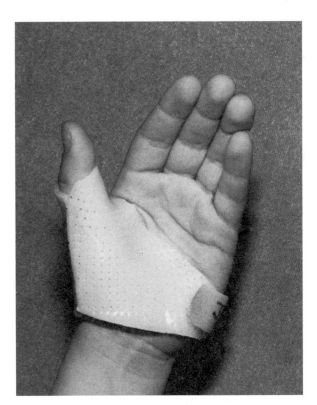

Figure **4.20**   The hardened splint is trimmed for comfort and maximum function

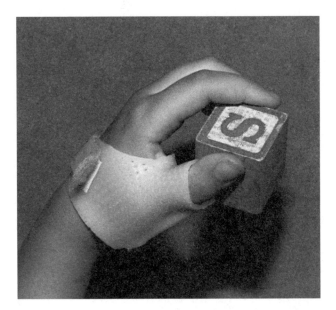

Figure **4.21**   The finished splint is secured onto the hand with one strap. It aligns the thumb into a position of function

## REFERENCES

This pattern is a modified version of the thumb spica splint produced by North Coast Medical. North Coast's splint blank is not available in pediatric sizes. Most manufacturers who sell splint blanks have a version of the thumb spica.

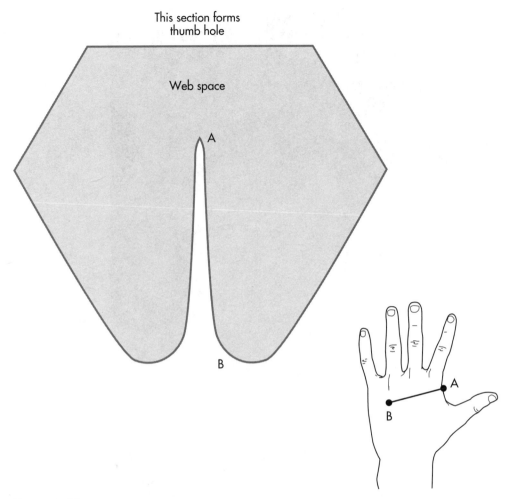

This section forms
thumb hole

Web space

A

B

A

B

Figure **4.22** Thumb Spica Splint

Copyright © 1998 by Therapy Skill Builders, a division of The Psychological Corporation/All rights reserved/
Laura Hogan and Tracey Uditsky, Pediatric Splinting/ISBN 0761615148/1-800-228-0752/This page is reproducible.

# Long Thumb Spica Splint

## Purpose

This splint is used to maintain the thumb in abduction and to support the thumb MP and CMC joints. This design also assists with aligning the wrist in a neutral position.

## Recommended Patient

This splint is not commonly used on infants or toddlers. It stabilizes the thumb and so does not allow dynamic thumb opposition. Therefore, it can interfere with functional use of the hand. It may be more commonly indicated for a child with juvenile rheumatoid arthritis (to rest and support a painful thumb) or post-op tendon transfers.

## Supplies and Materials

A solid or perforated thermoplastic material, either 1/8-inch, 1/12-inch, or 1/16-inch that is moderately rigid and has a moderate to high degree of conformability without too much stretch should be used. Recommended materials are elastics such as Aquaplast or soft Orfit, or plastic-rubbers such as Kay Splint Basic III, Preferred, or Polyflex II. In addition to the thermoplastic, you will need self-adhesive hook Velcro and either loop Velcro or Velfoam for the strapping. If you use a perforated thermoplastic material, you may need Aquaplast Ultra Thin Edging Material to finish the edges for comfort.

## Instructions for Splint or Pattern Making

You do not need a customized pattern to fabricate this splint. Measure the length from the child's thumb IP joint to the midpoint of the forearm. The width of the splint is determined by measuring the circumference of the forearm and dividing this number by two. These measurements are approximates only. Cut a rectangular piece of thermoplastic using the length and width measurements as instructed above. Heat your material and cut the rectangle. Generously round off the corners of the distal end of the splint (the end that will wrap around the thumb). The resulting shape should resemble a torpedo (see Figure 4.25 on page 105). With the patient's thumb abducted and the wrist in a neutral position, drape the heated material around the radial border of the forearm and wrist. Next, take the volar portion of the thumb piece and wrap it dorsally, overlapping the dorsal piece of the thumb. This creates a complete circumferential thumb post (Figure 4.23).

While the thermoplastic is drying, make sure the wrist is not in radial or ulnar deviation and that it is in neutral extension. The volar portion of the splint should support the thenar eminence but should not extend any farther into the palm than the thenar crease. Trim the thumb post just proximal to the thumb IP joint to allow full IP flexion (if that is desired). The width of the splint should end at midpoint both volarly and dorsally (Figure 4.24). Trim any excess, smooth edges with a heat gun, or apply Ultra Thin Edging as necessary. Apply wrist and forearm straps.

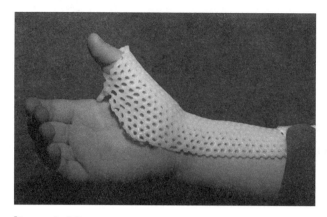

Figure **4.23** Volar view of the circumferential thumb post

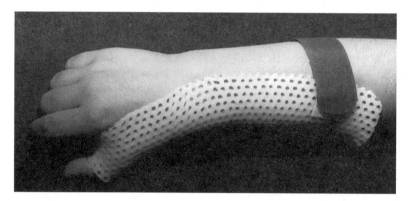

Figure **4.24** Trim the splint so it ends at the midpoint of the arm on both the dorsal and volar surfaces

## REFERENCES

This pattern is a modification of the North Coast Medical radial-based thumb spica splint.

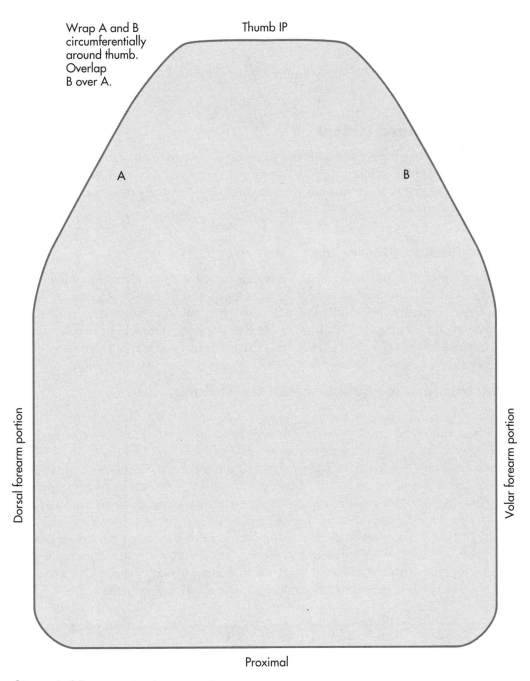

Wrap A and B circumferentially around thumb. Overlap B over A.

Thumb IP

A

B

Dorsal forearm portion

Volar forearm portion

Proximal

Figure **4.25** Long Thumb Spica Splint

Copyright © 1998 by Therapy Skill Builders, a division of The Psychological Corporation/All rights reserved/
Laura Hogan and Tracey Uditsky, Pediatric Splinting/ISBN 0761615148/1-800-228-0752/This page is reproducible.

## Volar Wrist Cock-Up Splint

### Purpose

This splint helps to prevent wrist drop and to support the wrist in neutral to slight extension.

### Recommended Patient

This splint design works best for the patient with extensor muscle weakness or absence or for the patient with only mildly increased flexor tone. It is not intended to be a wrist positioning splint for the patient with moderately or severely increased tone or significant wrist flexion.

### Supplies and Materials

Select a thermoplastic material that is at least moderately rigid and has a low level of stretch. It does not need to have a high degree of conformability. Recommended materials include elastics such as Aquaplast, plastic-rubbers such as Preferred, or rubbers such as Synergy or Orthoplast. In addition to the thermoplastic, you will need self-adhesive hook Velcro and loop Velcro or Velfoam for wrist and forearm strapping.

### Instructions for Splint or Pattern Making

Trace the child's hand on paper toweling. Draw a pattern that extends from the distal palmar transverse crease to half the length of the forearm (see Figure 4.27 on page 108). The wrist portion should remain on the volar surface only, then the splint widens laterally to extend half the distance up the radial and ulnar borders. Transfer your pattern to the selected thermoplastic material. Heat the material and cut out the pattern. Mold the splint, paying particular attention to ensure that the palmar portion conforms well to support the arches of the hand. It should clear the thenar crease so as not to block thumb opposition. Make sure the distal portion clears the distal palmar transverse crease so it does not interfere with MP flexion (Figure 4.26). Before the splint completely cools, position the wrist in the desired degree of extension (usually neutral to 15° extension). Once the splint is fully cool, add wrist and forearm strapping as needed.

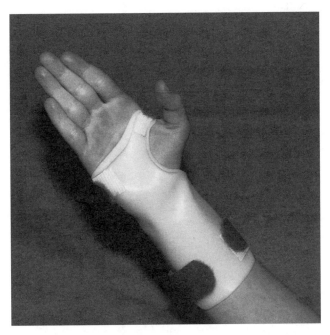

Figure **4.26**   Clear the distal palmar transverse crease to allow MP flexion

## REFERENCES

The authors designed the splint. It is a modification of the simple cock-up splint design in Malick, M. H. (1972). *Manual on static hand splinting*. Pittsburgh, PA: American Rehabilitation Educational Network.

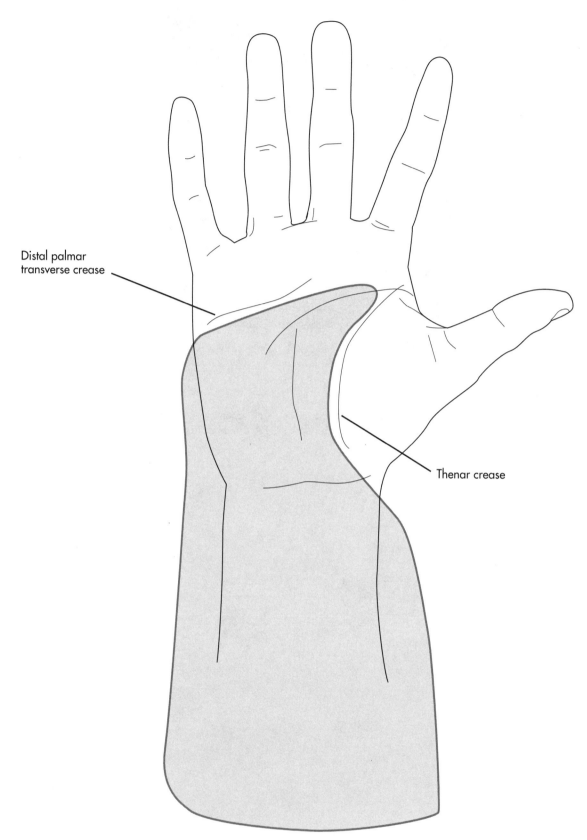

Distal palmar
transverse crease

Thenar crease

Figure **4.27** Volar Wrist Cock-Up Splint

Copyright © 1998 by Therapy Skill Builders, a division of The Psychological Corporation/All rights reserved/
Laura Hogan and Tracey Uditsky, Pediatric Splinting/ISBN 0761615148/1-800-228-0752/This page is reproducible.

# Volar Wrist Cock-Up Splint with Thumb-Abduction Loop

## Purpose

This splint can be used to prevent wrist drop and to support the wrist in neutral to slight extension while providing thumb abduction support to the thumb.

## Recommended Patient

This splint design may be selected when both the wrist and thumb are minimally involved and a resting-hand splint is more than is needed. It is a common mistake to "oversplint" when both the wrist and thumb joints are involved. This design incorporates a traditional static design with a semi-dynamic component (the neoprene thumb strap) added to facilitate functional hand use. This splint can be used for the child with cerebral palsy with mildly increased tone, brachial plexus injury, arthrogryposis, or other clinical conditions resulting in mild wrist flexion and thumb adduction.

## Supplies and Materials

Select a thermoplastic material that is at least moderately rigid and has a low level of stretch. It does not need to have a high degree of conformability. Elastic, plastic-rubber, or rubber materials work well (see volar wrist cock-up splint for specifics). You can use a 1/8-inch or 1/16-inch thermoplastic depending on the amount of increased tone or level of support your patient requires. You also will need a neoprene strap, regular loop Velcro, self-adhesive hook Velcro, and a sewing thread and needle.

## Instructions for Splint or Pattern Making

Follow the instructions for the volar wrist cock-up splint. Add a forearm and wrist strap. Cut a thin strip of neoprene to be used as the thumb abductor strap. Sew this strap onto the center of the wrist strap on the dorsum of the wrist, wrap it around the thumb in a figure-eight design, and then attach it on the radial volar surface using a regular loop to hook Velcro attachment. The figure-eight design is optional. You also can route the strap from the back of the wrist strap, through the web space, and across the thenar eminence. Then attach it to the radial volar surface (Figure 4.28). The tension on the neoprene thumb-abduction strap should be sufficient to maintain the thumb in abduction at rest while still allowing dynamic thumb opposition for function. Observe the dorsal side of the thumb to make sure the tension created by the neoprene strap is not causing hyperextension at the MP joint.

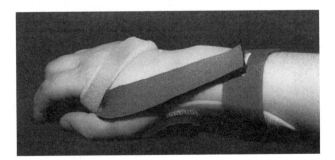

Figure **4.28** A thumb-abduction loop can be used with or without the strap proximal to the MP joints

**REFERENCES**

This design was developed by the authors.

## Volar Wrist Cock-Up Splint with Radial Bar

### Purpose

This splint is used to position the wrist in neutral alignment and wrist extension. It enables volitional active movement of the thumb and fingers.

### Recommended Patient

As with most types of cock-up splints, this splint works well to provide functional positioning for children with mild to moderate amounts of spasticity in the wrist and fingers who have some functional use of the thumb. It is also a good splint for children with muscular weakness because it is made with a minimal amount of material and is relatively light. Because it covers the volar aspect of the hand and forearm, it may not be the preferred splint for children who do a lot of weight-bearing on to their hands or forearms or those who spend a lot of time at the tabletop or computer keyboard.

### Supplies and Materials

Many types of materials can be used to make this splint. Something somewhat rigid and moderately conforming usually works well, but you might be able to get away with any thermoplastic in a pinch. We like 1/8-inch plastic-rubber materials such as Polyflex II, Preferred, and Kay Splint Basic II. For very small children and infants, use 1/16-inch material. In addition to the splinting material, you will need three straps.

### Instructions for Splint or Pattern Making

Trace the child's hand on a piece of paper. Mark the following anatomical landmarks: the MP joints of the index and little fingers and the ulnar and radial sides of the wrist joints. The pattern for this splint is easy to make (see Figure 4.31 on page 113). Do not let the instructions confuse you. This is another splint in which precise sizing is not required. Its borders can be rolled back or trimmed as needed.

Draw a line from point A to point B proximal to your MP landmarks at the distal palmar transverse crease. The start of the line (A) is about 1/2-inch from the ulnar side of the hand. It extends 1 to 2 inches past the radial side of the hand (B). At point B draw a line straight down to point C (it should be no farther than the web space). Draw a line from point A to point D (D is at the ulnar wrist joint 1/2-inch from the side of the hand). On the trace of your patient's hand, mark where the base of the thenar eminence would be. This is about half the distance from the thumb to the ulnar side of the wrist joint under the middle palmar crease. Now draw a curved line from point C around the thenar crease, through the base of the thenar eminence, to the radial side of the wrist joint as shown in the pattern. The wrist portion of the pattern flares out at the wrist joint. Make the length approximately two-thirds the length of your patient's forearm.

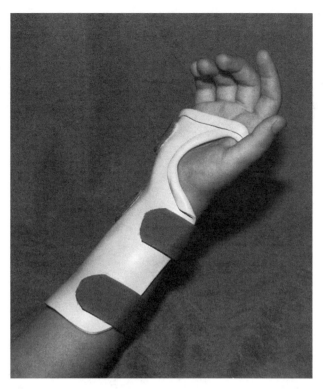

Figure **4.29** Volar view in which the material is rolled to clear the distal palmar transverse crease and the thenar crease

To fabricate the splint, form the radial bar around the child's hand. Roll the material as needed to clear the distal palmar transverse crease and the thenar crease (Figure 4.29). Form the forearm trough. Apply one strap from the radial bar across the back of the hand, one at the wrist, and one at the proximal portion of the forearm (Figure 4.30). There is not much surface area on the back of the radial bar to apply a strap. We recommend you attach that strap with a finger rivet instead of Velcro. In some cases, you may not need a strap on the radial bar at all.

**Important Note:** While you are forming the details of the hand, you may have the child's forearm in a supinated position but, when you finish forming the proximal trough, make sure that the hand is pronated and in the position to be worn or the rotation of the radius over the ulna in supination will cause the splint to fit incorrectly in pronation. If the child will cooperate, it is easiest to splint with the child's hand upright with the shoulder in external rotation. This principle applies to most splints that cover the wrist and forearm.

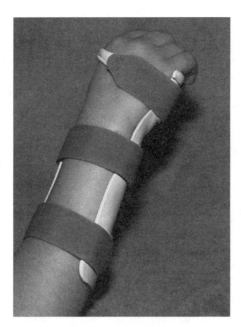

Figure **4.30** Completed splint with three straps. Due to the limited surface area on the radial bar, you may prefer to attach the strap with a rivet instead of Velcro

## REFERENCES

Splint blanks similar to this design can be obtained through Rehabilitation Division, Smith & Nephew, Inc.; North Coast Medical; and AliMed Inc.

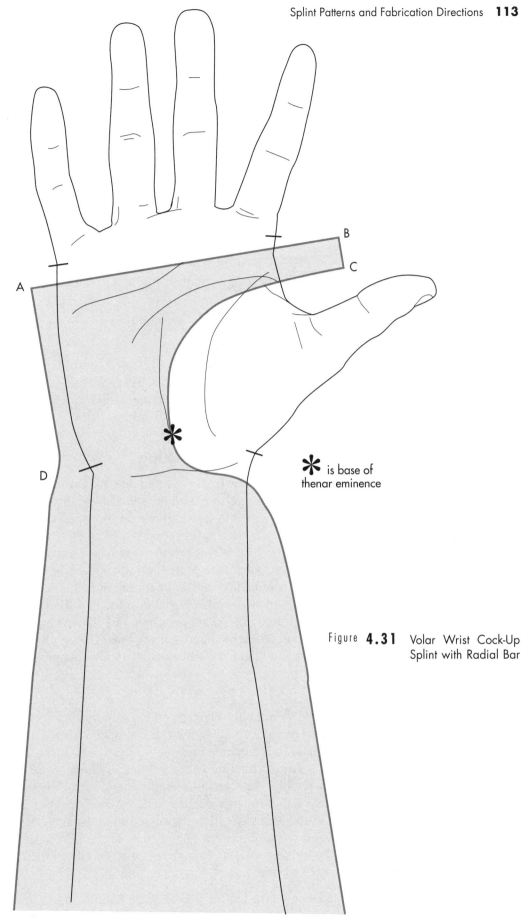

A

B

C

D

✱ is base of
thenar eminence

Figure **4.31** Volar Wrist Cock-Up
Splint with Radial Bar

Copyright © 1998 by Therapy Skill Builders, a division of The Psychological Corporation/All rights reserved/
Laura Hogan and Tracey Uditsky, Pediatric Splinting/ISBN 0761615148/1-800-228-0752/This page is reproducible.

## Volar Wrist Cock-Up Splint with Thumb Hole

### Purpose

This splint is used to properly align the wrist and place the hand in a position for function. This splint usually is worn during the day.

### Recommended Patient

This splint is ideal for children who have mild to moderate spasticity in the flexors of the wrist and fingers but not excessive spasticity in the flexors or adductors of the thumb. It also might be recommended for a child with some hypermobility of the thumb MP joint because the small opening around the thumb provides some support in a somewhat static position. Because it covers the volar surface of the forearm, it may not be indicated for children who do a lot of weight-bearing in a prone position or who sit and work at a tabletop or computer.

### Supplies and Materials

There are a variety of thermoplastic materials that work well for this splint. We recommend a material that is moderately rigid and with a moderate degree of stretch. You can use Spectrum, Aquaplast, or a similar material in either perforated or solid 1/8-inch or 3/32-inch thickness. Use Velcro loop and hook for straps.

### Instructions for Splint or Pattern Making

This is a pattern that is difficult to draw from your patient's anatomical landmarks. Either trace your patient's hand and draw a pattern with the same shape or place your patient's hand onto the pattern and compare for fit (see Figure 4.34 on page 116). If this pattern is the right size there will be about 1/2-inch surplus on all sides of your patient's hand, and the pattern will reach two-thirds of the way down the length of the forearm. Reproduce the pattern larger or smaller as needed. Precise sizing is not required for this splint. Its borders can be rolled back or trimmed. To make the thumb hole, mark the spot in the top portion of the splint slightly to the right for a left-hand splint and slightly to the left for a right-hand splint. Cut the thumb hole. (Cutting a hole can be done by using the end of a pencil to push up a mound of warm material at your mark. Snip off the mound and you have a hole about 1/4 inch in diameter. You can now easily enlarge the hole as needed with scissors.)

To fabricate, reheat the material (if necessary) and place it on the volar surface of your patient's hand. Put the child's thumb through the hole. Position the wrist in extension if possible (25° to 30° is good for functional activities). You may want to fabricate the hand portion first and then go back and fabricate the forearm trough. To form the hand portion of the splint, roll the edges around the thumb but not to the thenar crease as in a volar wrist cock-up splint with a radial bar. The thumb hole should be big enough to allow room for the thumb to move slightly, ensuring the material does not cut into the adductors or soft tissue in the web space. Roll the edges of the distal border proximal to the distal palmar transverse crease. Form the lateral edges around the sides of the hand at the web space and on the forearm. Attach three straps, and then decorate. The completed splint is shown in Figures 4.32 and 4.33.

Important Note: While you are forming the details of the hand, you may have the child's forearm in a supinated position. When you finish forming the proximal trough make sure

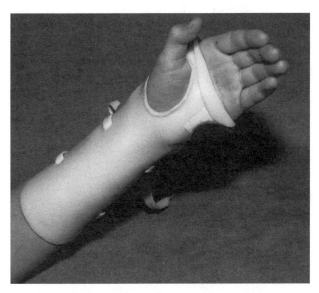

Figure **4.32** Volar view of the splint, demonstrating that the hole at the thumb is large enough for comfort and function

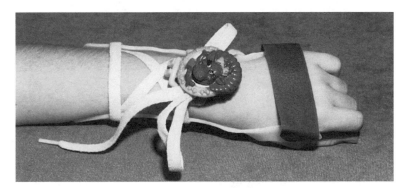

Figure **4.33** Completed splint, demonstrating the use of a shoelace and shoelace keeper for straps

the hand is pronated and in the position to wear the splint or the rotation of the radius over the ulna in supination will cause the splint to fit incorrectly in pronation. If the child will cooperate, it is easiest to splint with the hand upright and the shoulder in external rotation.

The splint is just another version of the familiar wrist cock-up splint. One of the design features, solid plastic around the opening of the thumb, may make this a preferred splint for children with moderate to severe spasticity but who still have potential for functional use. You can modify this splint by making the thumb hole larger and rolling it clear of the thenar eminence for use on children with more spasticity in the thumb. This design of the wrist cock-up splint with thumb hole allows more room to attach straps than the wrist cock-up splint with radial bar.

### REFERENCES

Splint blanks similar to this design can be obtained through Rehabilitation Division, Smith & Nephew, Inc.; North Coast Medical; and AliMed Inc.

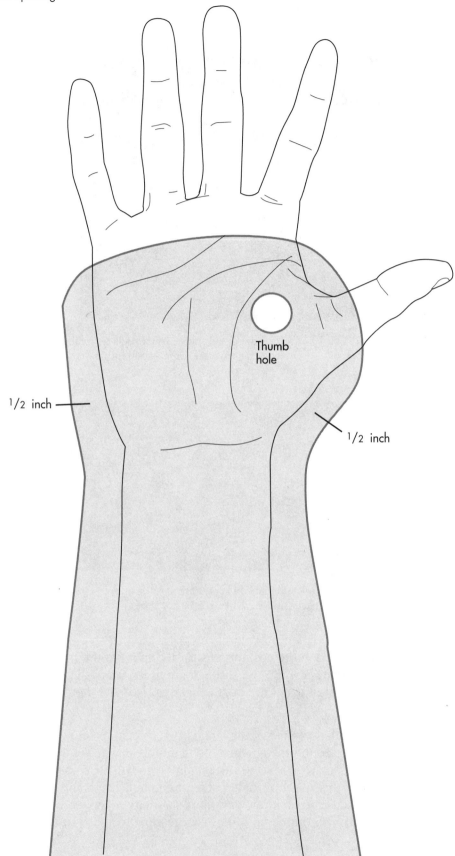

1/2 inch

Thumb
hole

1/2 inch

Figure **4.34** Volar Wrist Cock-Up Splint with Thumb Hole

Copyright © 1998 by Therapy Skill Builders, a division of The Psychological Corporation/All rights reserved/
Laura Hogan and Tracey Uditsky, Pediatric Splinting/ISBN 0761615148/1-800-228-0752/This page is reproducible.

# Dorsal Wrist Cock-Up Splint

## Purpose

This splint can be used to prevent wrist drop and to maintain the wrist in neutral extension. It is indicated for wrist immobilization or support.

## Recommended Patient

This dorsal design leaves the volar surface of the forearm free for uninhibited sensory input and weight bearing. This splint is recommended for patients who are not yet ambulatory and therefore spend a great deal of time prone on the floor with potential for the volar surface of the forearm to make contact with the floor. This design also is recommended for patients who require a cock-up splint but spend time sitting at a tabletop participating in functional activities such as writing, typing, etc., with the forearm bearing weight on the tabletop.

## Supplies and Materials

Select a thermoplastic material that is at least moderately rigid but does not have a high degree of stretch. Recommended materials include elastics such as Aquaplast or plastic-rubbers such as Polyflex II. You also will need self-adhesive hook Velcro and regular loop Velcro or Velfoam for strapping.

## Instructions for Splint or Pattern Making

This is a pattern that is difficult to draw from your patient's anatomical landmarks. The total length is from the proximal palmar transverse crease to two-thirds the length of the forearm. The width is about half the total circumference of the patient's forearm (see Figure 4.37 on page 119). To estimate the appropriate pattern size, we recommend that you have several pre-cut prototype patterns (made from Naugahyde) in varying sizes available to try on your patients. Place the prototype pattern on your patient's hand to assess for fit. Reduce or enlarge the pattern as needed.

Once you have selected an appropriately sized pattern, trace it on the thermoplastic material of your choice. Heat the material and cut out your pattern. If necessary, reheat the material before fabrication. Once the material is fully warmed, place the patient's extended fingers through the distal cutout so that the distal-most portion of the splint becomes a volar bar. This will be used to create a palmar arch support. Make sure the straight edge is the distal-most point, and the edge with the bump is pointing toward the wrist (Figure 4.35).

The remainder of the splint will then lie on the dorsum of the patient's wrist and forearm. It should be allowed to drape around the forearm, ending at mid-position (Figure 4.36). As the material is drying, make sure the wrist remains in neutral extension and is not deviated either radially or ulnarly. At the wrist, fold the radial and ulnar borders dorsally for additional strength and support. Conform the palmar bar slightly into the arch of the hand and make sure it is not interfering with MP flexion (it should clear the distal palmar transverse crease). Allow the splint to cool completely. Attach a strap to the proximal end of the forearm portion.

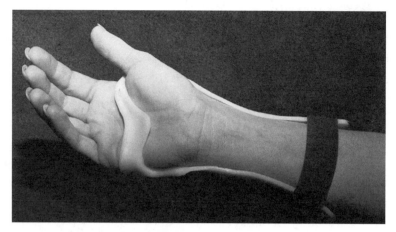

Figure **4.35** Volar view of the dorsal wrist cock-up splint

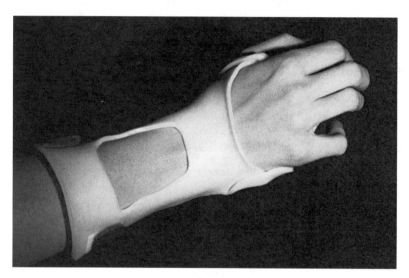

Figure **4.36** Dorsal view of the dorsal wrist cock-up splint

## REFERENCES

This splint design is found in North Coast Medical and Rehabilitation Division, Smith & Nephew Inc. catalogs.

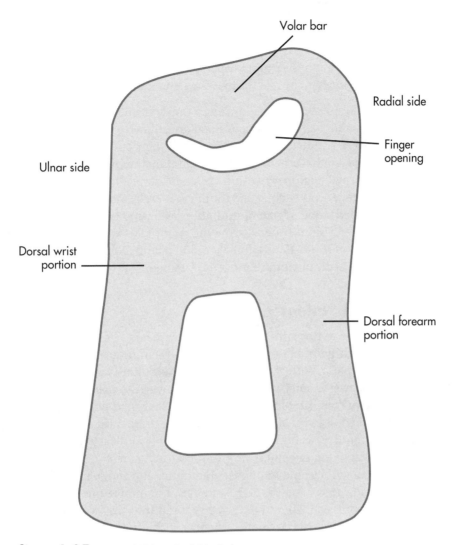

Volar bar

Radial side

Finger opening

Ulnar side

Dorsal wrist portion

Dorsal forearm portion

Figure **4.37** Dorsal Wrist Cock-Up Splint

Copyright © 1998 by Therapy Skill Builders, a division of The Psychological Corporation/All rights reserved/
Laura Hogan and Tracey Uditsky, Pediatric Splinting/ISBN 0761615148/1-800-228-0752/This page is reproducible.

## Circumferential Wrist-Positioning Splint

### Purpose

The splint is worn to align the hand properly and to progressively increase wrist and finger range of motion. It may also "relax" the hand and arm.

The benefits of this splint are gained through the circumferential design with a pronounced palmar arch. The wrist and hand are aligned into a neutral, functional position that does not stretch the muscles beyond their current maximum range. The splint was developed using a neurodevelopmental treatment frame of reference. The emphasis is on normal alignment within the comfortable limits of range of the child, using key points of control such as the thumb and arches to control the hand. Typical results have included some degree of inhibition of spasticity of the wrist, thumb, and fingers. Usually after a short time wearing the splint (1–4 weeks), the child will gain wrist and finger range of motion. New splints should be fabricated within the child's new comfortable ranges until maximum range is obtained.

### Recommended Patient

The optimal benefits of this splint will be achieved when used with a child who has had a recent injury resulting in neuromuscular impairment. It also works well with children who have cerebral palsy, both mild and severe. This splint is recommended for children with frequent upper-extremity muscle spasms because the material bends with the child. This makes it more comfortable to wear than a typical rigid resting-hand splint. The more severe the wrist flexion contracture a child has, the more difficult it may be for you to fabricate this splint. Because this splint is comfortable and easy to wear, it may be a good choice for children living in centers or group homes where caregivers are busy. With the splint on, children will be able to oppose the thumb and index finger, but because the palm is covered all the way up to the MP creases, fine-motor manipulative skills will be restricted. This splint also will reduce sensory input into the extremity. Because of its circumferential design, it is extremely difficult for children to remove this splint by themselves. Based on the size of your patient and the degree of spasticity, it may be difficult for the caregiver to put on by himself as well.

### Supplies and Materials

Use 1/12-inch micro-perforated soft Orfit or a similar thin perforated material and Velcro loop and hook for straps. Therapy putty to cover the ulnar styloid process or other bony prominences during fabrication is highly recommended.

### Instructions for Splint or Pattern Making

Measure the width of the child's hand at the MP heads and about two-thirds of the way up the forearm. Add 1 inch to the widest measurement. This will be the width of your splint. The length is the distance from the MP heads to two-thirds the length of the forearm. To locate the position for the thumb hole, measure the distance from the MP head of the index finger (A) to the MP head of the thumb (B). Make your mark for the thumb hole at that measurement, straight down from the top of the splinting material, in one-third the width of the splint (see Figure 4.42 on page 124). To fabricate the splint, first cut the thumb hole. To do this, heat the material and use the end of a

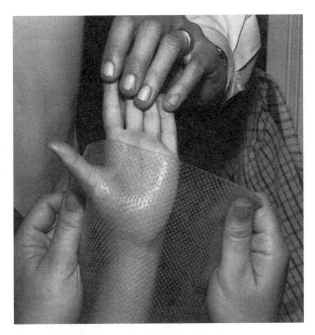

Figure **4.38**  Start to fabricate this splint by placing the material over the thumb through the hole. It helps to have someone extend the fingers whenever possible

pencil to push up a mound of warm material at your mark. Snip off the mound and you will have a hole about 1/4 inch in diameter. Since this material cools quickly, reheat it to continue fabricating.

**Important Tips:** For this splint, the position of the hand is important. Spend a few minutes with your patient prior to fabrication. Work to inhibit tone, relax the hand, and passively range the joints. Place a small piece of therapy putty directly onto the patient's skin over the ulnar styloid process or any other prominent bony landmarks. You will be fabricating directly over the putty. It will not affect the outcome of the splint and is easily removed when the thermoplastic material has cooled. The bump in the material will inhibit pressure breakdown at that spot. During fabrication it is helpful to have a second person available to assist.

Place the warm material over the thumb through the hole. The longer side of the material covers the volar surface of the hand (Figure 4.38). Bring the two lateral edges of the splint together over the dorsum. Pinch them together to hold the splint on the patient while you align the wrist (Figure 4.39).

While you form the arches of the palm, pull the thumb hole down to the thumb MP and trim or roll the distal border of the material to just proximal of the MP creases (Figure 4.40). Stroke the volar surface of the splint in a distal to proximal direction to keep the wrist crease smooth and conformed. Because a child's hand is small, it is usually recommended that the therapist position his or her thumb into the palm, maintaining the arches and wrist position until the splint material has cooled. Do not overwork the thermoplastic material in the palm or the perforations will open up too widely, weakening the integrity of the splint. When the material has cooled, unsnap the pinched material on the dorsum of the forearm and remove the splint from the child. Trim the lateral edges so

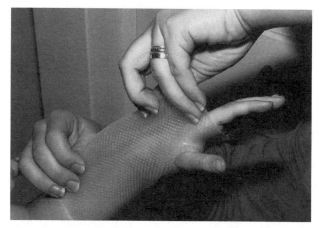

Figure **4.39** Gently pinch the lateral edges of the splint on the dorsum before you form the arches of the palm

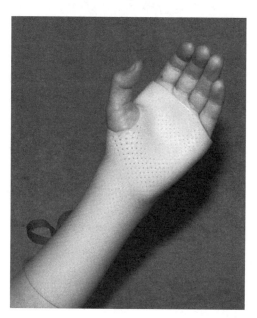

Figure **4.40** Unlike a volar wrist cock-up splint, the distal border of the splint supports the MP heads and extends to just proximal of the MP creases. The thenar eminence is covered, the thumb CMC and MP joints are immobilized

that when in place, the circumferential splint wraps around the forearm, leaving just a 1/2-inch to 3/4-inch gap on the dorsum. (The gap can be up to 1 inch for larger children and adolescents.) Apply three straps: one proximal, one distal, and one over the dorsum of the wrist, or use an alternate strapping method (Figure 4.41).

**Important Note:** Remember, this is not a wrist cock-up splint. The distal border should extend all the way to the MP creases, and the thenar eminence should be supported (covered) by the splint. Because of the common characteristic of tight thumb adductors

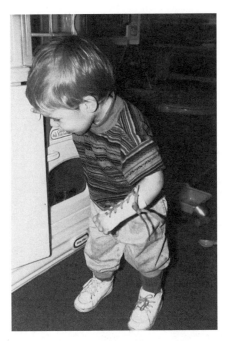

Figure **4.41**  A completed splint utilizing a shoelace instead of straps to prevent this little boy from removing his splint independently at inappropriate times

in children with spastic cerebral palsy, be sure to check the area around the thumb for comfort and absence of pressure marks. This splint often has such dramatic effects on the range of motion of the upper extremity that the splint needs to be refabricated several times to maximize the amount of range available to the child as treatment progresses. Because you are using a piece of thermoplastic material with 100% memory, you can throw the material back in the splinting pan to refabricate the splint or to start over if you make a mistake fabricating the splint. Orfit can be hard to splint with until you get used to it. Try to be patient and look for someone to help you if possible.

**REFERENCES**

The authors modified the design of this splint, provided by a North Coast Medical Supplies sales representative in 1994, to better fit pediatric hands.

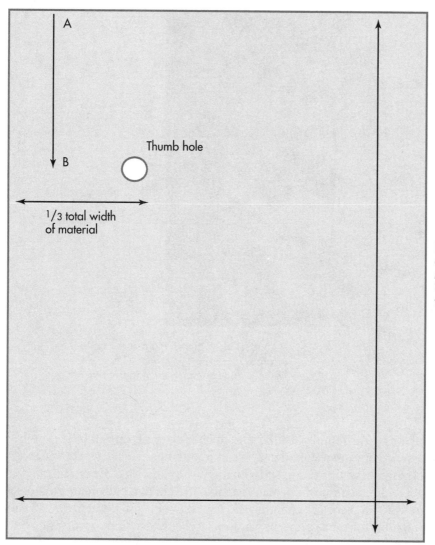

A

Thumb hole

B

1/3 total width
of material

Length equals the
distance of the
MP heads to
2/3 the length of
the forearm.

Width equals the widest
circumference of the hand
or forearm plus 1".

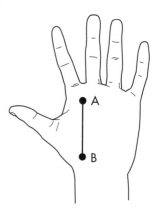

A

B

Figure **4.42** Circumferential Wrist-Positioning Splint

Copyright © 1998 by Therapy Skill Builders, a division of The Psychological Corporation/All rights reserved/
Laura Hogan and Tracey Uditsky, Pediatric Splinting/ISBN 0761615148/1-800-228-0752/This page is reproducible.

## Wrist Gauntlet Splint

### Purpose

Use this splint to immobilize the wrist while providing proper positioning and rest. This splint's distal edge is proximal to the transverse arches and therefore allows free movement of the MPs and grasp.

### Recommended Patient

Customarily this splint is used with children who have juvenile rheumatoid arthritis or other inflammatory conditions to provide support and protection during a painful flare-up. It may be used post-surgically, as well, if immobilization of the wrist is necessary. This splint is not the preferred splint for children with neurological impairments. (Refer to the circumferential wrist positioning splint pattern for a similar splint designed to provide positioning and increase range of motion of children with moderate and severe spasticity.)

### Supplies and Materials

Because this splint has a circumferential design, it should be fabricated from a flexible, thin elastic material such as 1/12-inch micro-perforated soft Orfit or 1/16-inch Aquaplast super-perforated. Three straps are needed. Therapy putty may be used to pre-pad the ulnar styloid process or any other bony prominences if needed.

### Instructions for Splint or Pattern Making

This splint is made from a simple pattern (see Figure 4.45 on page 127). The length of the material to be used is equivalent to the length of the child's hand from the MP head of the index finger to two-thirds of the way up the forearm. The width of the splint is the widest measurement of the hand or mid-forearm plus 1 inch. With these two measurements, draw a pattern that resembles a house with a low-sloped roof. Cut a hole 1/2 inch to 1 1/2 inches below the "peak of the roof" for the thumb. (The distance depends on the size of the child's hand. You don't need to be too precise because you can trim and roll down the distal edge of this splint once it is formed.) To cut the thumb hole, heat the material, use the end of a pencil to push up a mound of warm material at your mark, and snip off the mound for a hole about 1/4 inch in diameter.

Place the heated material over the child's hand, starting with the thumb through the hole. Drape the material around the volar and dorsal surfaces and pinch it together on the ulnar dorsal side of the hand. Conform the material to the wrist and forearm, making sure you have the hand positioned in the desired alignment. Roll back the thumb hole. Roll back the distal border of the splint to clear the distal palmar transverse crease. When the material has almost cooled, unsnap the pinched edges and remove the splint. Trim the edges of the splint leaving a 1-inch to 1 1/2-inch gap on the ulnar dorsal aspect of the hand. Apply three straps. The completed splint is shown in Figures 4.43 and 4.44.

**Important Note:** This splint protects the wrist well during an inflammatory phase a child may be experiencing. It is important to pull the splint open thoroughly to enable the child to get in and out of it. If the child tries to don and doff this splint independently, or

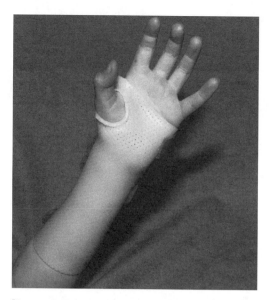

Figure **4.43** The distal border of the splint clears the distal palmar transverse crease and the thumb opening is large enough to allow functional use of the hand

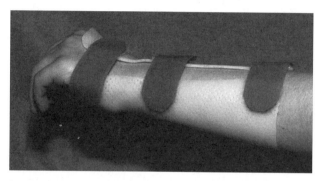

Figure **4.44** The opening of the splint on the dorsum is displaced ulnarly and is 1 to 1½ inches wide

the caretaker does not open the splint far enough, the child may bump the inflamed wrist on the sides and complain of pain. The design of this splint makes it a little difficult for a child to don and doff unassisted. If your patient needs to be independent with this skill, you may opt to make the gap on the dorsum larger or select a wrist cock-up splint with thumb hole.

### REFERENCES

Splint blanks similar to this design are available through North Coast Medical.

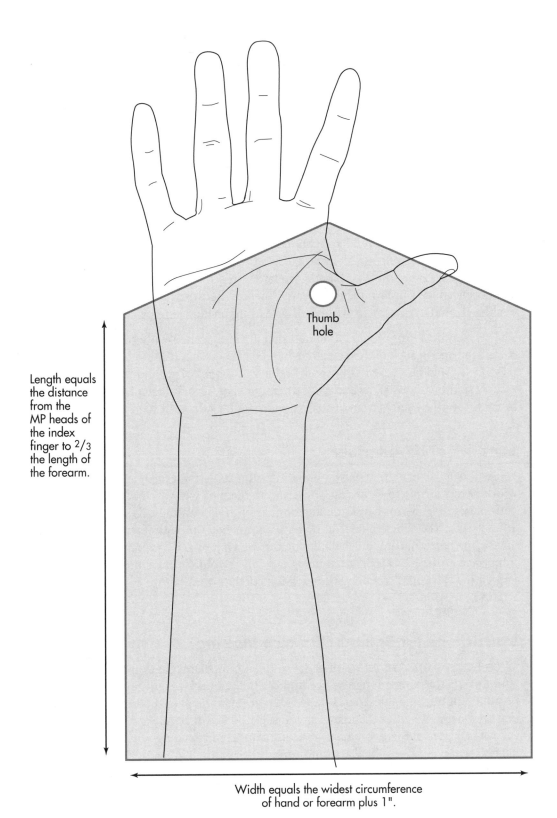

Length equals the distance from the MP heads of the index finger to $2/3$ the length of the forearm.

Thumb hole

Width equals the widest circumference of hand or forearm plus 1".

Figure **4.45** Wrist Gauntlet Splint

Copyright © 1998 by Therapy Skill Builders, a division of The Psychological Corporation/All rights reserved/ Laura Hogan and Tracey Uditsky, Pediatric Splinting/ISBN 0761615148/1-800-228-0752/This page is reproducible.

## Serpentine Splint

### Purpose

This splint is used to inhibit thumb adduction, position the wrist in neutral alignment, and facilitate forearm supination. The serpentine splint is not completely static. It provides dynamic support without completely blocking wrist extension or thumb opposition, thereby enabling functional use of the hand. This splint can also be used as a "weaning" splint to transition from a static splint to no splint at all.

### Recommended Patient

This splint is used most commonly for children with cerebral palsy or other neurological conditions that result in mildly increased muscle tone. It also can be used with children who have mildly decreased muscle tone (such as Down syndrome) or arthrogryposis. The splint is intended to be worn during functional activities. The serpentine splint can be a nice adjunct to therapy because it is not totally static. It enables dynamic movement while still providing needed support and alignment.

The serpentine splint often is tolerated socially and cosmetically by children because of its "non-medical" look (especially when fabricated in a bright-colored thermoplastic). It is also a good choice for children who have a history of splint intolerance secondary to rashes, skin breakdown, or excessive sweating. The serpentine splint is very cost-effective because it only requires a small strip of material for fabrication.

### Supplies and Materials

You will need a strip of an elastic-based thermoplastic material such as Aquaplast. The width of this strip will be about 1 inch and the length will vary according to the size of your patient's forearm. Until you are familiar with fabricating this splint, allow yourself at least 16 to 18 inches in length. If you want an exact measurement, use a cloth measuring tape. Starting on the palm below the ring finger (proximal to the distal palmar transverse crease), wrap the measuring tape up the child's extremity as though you were fabricating the splint (see the following instructions and Figure 4.49 on page 131 for how to wrap the splint).

### Instructions for Splint or Pattern Making

Cut a 1-inch strip of splinting material to the appropriate length. Heat it until soft. If your splint pan is not long enough to accommodate the entire length of the material, heat a portion of it until pliable, then fold it so the rest can be placed beside the first part. If you are unsure whether the material you selected is self-bonding, place a paper towel in the water between the two halves to keep them from touching. Once the entire strip is heated, remove it from the water and roll it into a long log. Form the splint by wrapping the material around the child's hand and forearm in the direction of supination.

When forming, pull (stretch) the material slightly, ensuring that the material conforms to the skin. It is this contact that allows the serpentine design of the splint to passively stretch the child's forearm into supination while inhibiting thumb adduction and aligning the wrist. Begin by placing the end of the strip on the palm proximal to the distal palmar transverse crease below the ring finger (Figure 4.46). Wrap the material ulnarly and

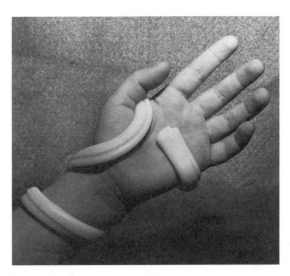

Figure **4.46** A volar view of correct splint placement

continue around the dorsum of the hand proximal to the MPs into the thumb web space. From the web space, follow the line of the thenar crease (remember you need good skin contact) to the base of the third metacarpal and make a U-turn, heading back in a radial direction under the base of the thumb to the dorsal aspect of the wrist (Figure 4.47). Continue spiraling the material two-thirds of the way up the forearm, stretching slightly and supinating as you go. Usually two to three spirals are sufficient. Keep in mind that the more spirals in the splint, the more force the splint will have to provide supination.

You can easily make several modifications to this splint. If the log-roll technique does not seem to "grip" the forearm well enough to achieve supination, or the splint shifts significantly on the forearm, you can tri-fold the material rather than roll it. This will result in a flat strip versus a rolled log and will be more stable against the arm. We prefer using this flat strip rather than a rolled log. Another variation to achieve greater supination calls for the attachment of a 1-inch wide strip of neoprene to the proximal end of the splint (use a rivet or Velcro). Continue to spiral the neoprene just proximal to the elbow joint. Attach the neoprene to itself with Velcro, forming an arm cuff (Figure 4.48). If the goal is to achieve greater supination, remember to form the splint and allow it to harden while the patient's forearm is maintained in the desired position. A common mistake is to form the splint while the patient's forearm is pronated rather than supinated.

A short serpentine is fabricated the same way as the standard version but stops at the base of the thumb. It does not spiral up the forearm. This short version is used for thumb positioning and inhibits minimal thumb adduction. It does not affect wrist position or forearm supination.

Another modification is to add a thumb post to the portion wrapped around the thenar eminence (as mentioned in the referenced article). This modification would be used to further inhibit thumb adduction in children with slightly higher muscle tone in the thumb adductors.

To remove the splint, start at the proximal end and "uncoil" the serpentine from the forearm in an ulnar to radial direction. Once you have uncoiled the spirals, simply slide the splint off the hand. To put the splint on, just reverse this process. Slide the fingers and

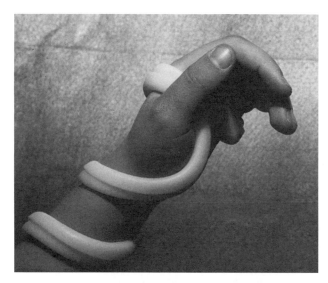

Figure **4.47** Correct placement from a radial view

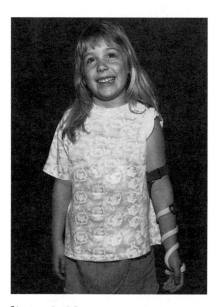

Figure **4.48** Completed splint with an additional neoprene strap to facilitate increased forearm supination

hand (but not the thumb) through the distal ulnar cuff. Make sure the U-turn is making good contact with the thenar eminence crease. Coil your spirals up the forearm in a radial to ulnar direction.

## REFERENCES

Thompson-Rangel, T. (1991, September 20). The mystery of the serpentine splints. *Occupational Therapy Forum*, 4–6.

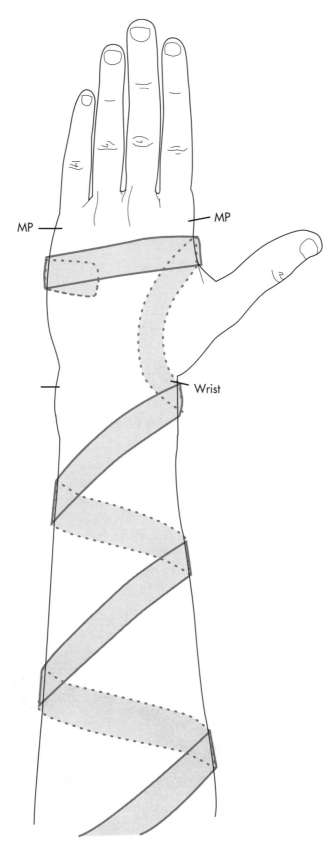

Figure **4.49** Serpentine Splint (Dorsal view)

Copyright © 1998 by Therapy Skill Builders, a division of The Psychological Corporation/All rights reserved/
Laura Hogan and Tracey Uditsky, Pediatric Splinting/ISBN 0761615148/1-800-228-0752/This page is reproducible.

## Resting-Hand Splint

### Purpose

This splint typically is used to prevent or decrease deformities in the wrist and fingers. It places the hand in a static, functional resting position.

### Recommended Patient

This splint can be used with a variety of diagnoses. It commonly is recommended for the child with cerebral palsy who has spastic wrist and finger flexors. It also can be used to rest the hand of a child with muscular weakness and position it so that deformities are prevented or minimized. Because the splint covers so much surface area of the hand, there can be no functional hand use while wearing the splint. For this reason, many therapists recommend this splint for nighttime use and a more functional hand splint to be worn during the day.

### Supplies and Materials

Because there is little contour needed on this splint, a rubber or plastic-rubber material works well. An elastic material also can be used. If your patient has spasticity, you probably will want to select a material that is rather rigid. Material 1/8-inch thick usually is sufficient. You will need at least three straps.

### Instructions for Splint or Pattern Making

There are numerous variations of this pattern from which to choose. We have found that this one works well for children. To make the pattern, first trace the child's hand. Mark the following anatomical landmarks: the web space (A), the ulnar and radial sides of the wrist, and between the index and middle fingers at the proximal palmar transverse crease (B). To make your pattern, start at the ulnar wrist joint, 1/4 inch to 1/2 inch from the tracing of the child's hand, and draw up and around the fingers to the radial side of the hand. Draw your line straight down through the web space (A) to the radial side of the wrist joint. Continue to curve the thumb piece as shown in Figure 4.53 (page 135) and up to the proximal palmar transverse crease (B). The wrist portion of the

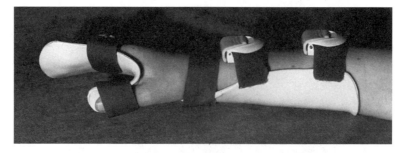

Figure **4.50**   Lateral view demonstrating good contact at the web space, the thumb in opposition to the fingers

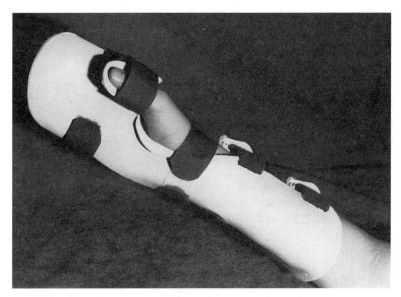

Figure **4.51** Material is rolled away from the thenar eminence to increase comfort

pattern flares out at the wrist joint. Make the length about two-thirds the length of your patient's forearm.

To fabricate the splint, trace the pattern on the material after trying it on your patient's hand for fit. The thumb piece contours around the thumb. Make sure the web space has good contact (Figure 4.50). On the volar surface, slightly roll the radial side of the material away from the thenar eminence to increase comfort (Figure 4.51). Apply a strap around the thumb. Apply three more straps, one across the fingers near the MPs, one at the wrist, and one at the proximal portion of the forearm. Figure 4.52 shows a completed splint. A fifth strap was added to this splint so the diaper clips could be used.

**Important Note:** While you are forming the details of the hand, you may have the child's forearm in a supinated position. But when you finish forming the proximal forearm trough, make sure that the hand is pronated and in the position the splint will be worn. If the child's forearm is not in a pronated position when you form the thermoplastic material on the forearm, the rotation of the radius over the ulna in supination will cause the splint to fit incorrectly.

If you are splinting a child with spasticity and your goal is to increase the range of motion at the wrist or fingers, it is better to position the child in a submaximal range, have the child wear the splint for an appropriate length of time per day, and then refabricate the splint if substantial range increases are obtained. Using this philosophy, your initial splint may be fabricated in slight wrist flexion or the finger pan curved to allow finger flexion.

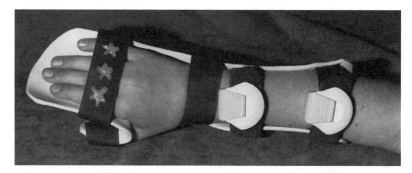

Figure **4.52** Completed splint demonstrating the use of diaper clips to keep a child from removing the splint independently at inappropriate times

## REFERENCES

This splint design, and a similar design frequently referred to as a resting pan or a functional positioning splint, is found in Rehabilitation Division, Smith & Nephew, Inc.; North Coast Medical; Sammons Preston and AliMed Inc.

AliMed Inc. sells pre-fabricated Comfy™ Splints for the wrist and elbow. They are padded, adjustable splints that come with washable terry-cloth covers in several fun colors. The prices range from $95 to $140 plus shipping and handling.

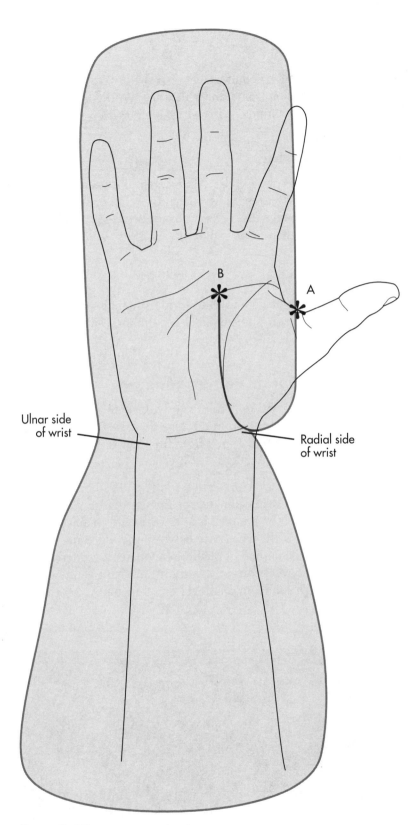

Ulnar side
of wrist

Radial side
of wrist

B

A

Figure **4.53**  Resting-Hand Splint

Copyright © 1998 by Therapy Skill Builders, a division of The Psychological Corporation/All rights reserved/
Laura Hogan and Tracey Uditsky, Pediatric Splinting/ISBN 0761615148/1-800-228-0752/This page is reproducible.

# Mitt Splint

## Purpose

This splint is used to provide a comfortable resting position for the wrist and fingers. The pan usually is curved to allow some finger flexion, and the thumb is in extension rather than abduction and opposition like the resting-hand splint.

## Recommended Patient

This splint is recommended for children with cerebral palsy who have spastic wrist and finger flexors. It can be used to increase range of motion or to rest the hand and position it so that deformities are prevented or minimized. Because the splint covers so much surface area of the hand, there is no functional hand use while wearing the splint.

## Supplies and Materials

A semi rigid or rigid material such as Multiform, Aquaplast, or Clinic is recommended, usually in 1/8-inch thickness. Three wide (1 1/2-inch to 2-inch), soft straps also are needed.

## Instructions for Splint or Pattern Making

There is no pattern easier to make than the one for the mitt splint. Simply trace the child's hand and draw a big circle around it (see Figure 4.55 on page 138). The lateral edges of the splint are 1/2 inch to 1 inch from the trace of the hand; the length of the splint is about two-thirds the length of the forearm.

To fabricate the splint, mold the pan portion to the child's hand with the wrist positioned in a comfortable amount of extension and the fingers slightly flexed. The thumb should be extended slightly. While the material is still warm and pliable, take a dowel or pencil and push the material up at the web space between the index finger and thumb to create a cradle for the thumb. This method of pushing the material up tends to keep the thumb in the splint better than other versions of this splint that have a cut at the web space separating the thumb portion from the finger pan portion. Apply two straps over

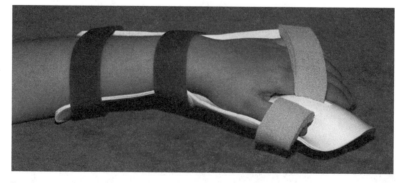

Figure **4.54** Completed splint demonstrating how to attach the strap over the thumb and fingers

the forearm and one over the thumb and fingers. We recommend using a rotary punch and a utility knife to make two slots in the material. The thumb strap has its first attachment on the volar surface. It wraps over the thumb, down the first slot, and up the second slot. Continue the strap over the finger pan and attach it with Velcro on the volar surface (Figure 4.54). You may want to trim a wide strap at the thumb so it is sufficient to secure the thumb but not too bulky.

**Important Note:** As with most splints that cover the wrist and forearm, you must be careful to fabricate the forearm trough in a pronated position (the position in which it will be worn). If you finish the splint while the forearm is supinated, the rotation of the radius over the ulna will cause the splint to fit incorrectly in pronation.

### REFERENCES

A modified version of this splint called a resting pan mitt splint is available through Rehabilitation Division, Smith & Nephew, Inc.; North Coast Medical; and AliMed Inc.

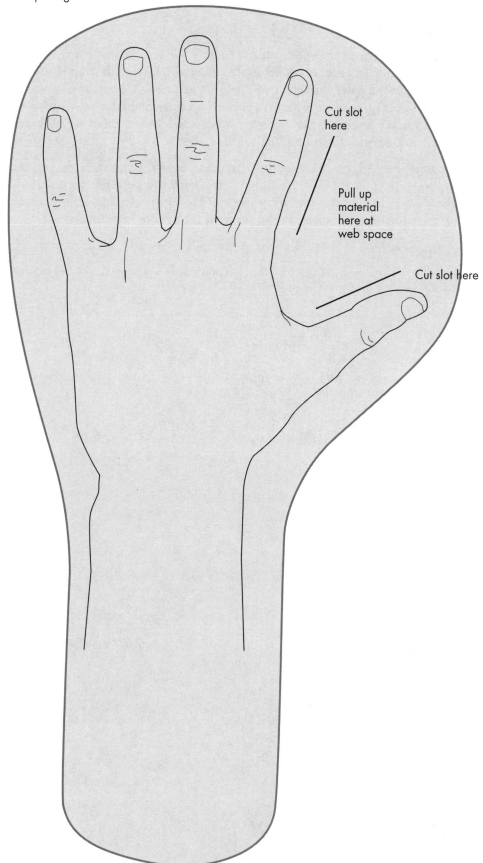

Cut slot
here

Pull up
material
here at
web space

Cut slot here

Figure **4.55** Mitt Splint

Copyright © 1998 by Therapy Skill Builders, a division of The Psychological Corporation/All rights reserved/
Laura Hogan and Tracey Uditsky, Pediatric Splinting/ISBN 0761615148/1-800-228-0752/This page is reproducible.

## Volar Anti-Spasticity Splint

### Purpose

This splint helps to position the hand in the reflex-inhibiting position of wrist extension, finger extension, and finger and thumb abduction. This design maintains the palmar arch and theoretically reduces muscle tone.

### Recommended Patient

This pattern is recommended for patients with severe hypertonicity resulting from cerebral palsy, traumatic brain injuries, or other neurological conditions resulting in abnormal muscle tone. The same pattern can be used to fabricate either a volar-based or dorsal-based forearm piece.

### Supplies and Materials

Select a 1/8-inch thermoplastic material that is rigid and has very little stretch. Because this splint is fabricated on patients with severe hypertonicity, you must use a material you have control over. Recommended materials include rubbers such as Orthoplast or Ezeform. If your splinting skills are at an intermediate to advanced level, you may be successful with Aquaplast materials, with the exception of Aquaplast ProDrape-T. In addition, you will need self-adhesive hook Velcro and regular loop Velcro or Velfoam for a forearm strap.

### Instructions for Splint or Pattern Making

Using paper toweling, trace the patient's hand with the fingers and thumb in maximum abduction. You do not need to trace between each individual finger or between the index finger and thumb. The length of the splint should be two-thirds the length of the forearm and the width should be sufficient to cover one-half the forearm circumference on both the radial and ulnar borders (see Figure 4.57 on page 141).

Transfer your pattern to the selected thermoplastic material, heat, and cut. Form the splint to the patient's extremity with the wrist in neutral to slight extension, the fingers and thumb in maximum abduction, and slight flexion at the PIPs and distal interphalangeals (DIPs). To achieve this slightly flexed position of all digits, you may form the hand portion over an appropriately sized ball. The ball helps achieve an overall spherical position. Before the material cools, use a dowel or other object to bring the material up between each finger and between the thumb and index finger (Figure 4.56). These ridges create individual finger troughs and maintain the fingers and thumb in optimal abduction. Cradle the forearm portion around the extremity and make sure that good palmar contact has been achieved to maintain palmar arches. Cool the splint, finish any rough edges, and attach a forearm strap. No additional straps should be necessary but assess the finished product and add additional strapping if needed.

If you are using this pattern for a dorsal-based forearm portion, follow the above pattern design directions but in addition to tracing the hand, mark the MP joints of both the second and fifth digits as well as the thumb (Figure 4.57). After heating the material, cut out the MP openings for the fingers and thumb by slitting the heated material with

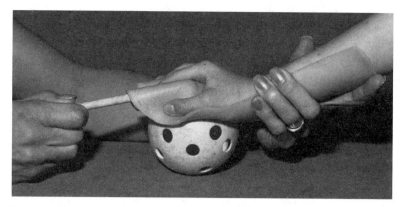

Figure **4.56** Use a dowel to bring the material up between each finger

scissors. Place the fingers through the pre-cut MP opening and the thumb through the pre-cut thumb opening. Next, place the splint on the dorsum of the forearm, allowing it to drape around the radial and ulnar aspects of the forearm. Cradle the thumb portion around the thumb to create a slight trough. Mold the volar finger pan with the fingers in slight PIP and DIP flexion. Again, if desired, use an appropriately sized ball to help achieve this slight spherical position of the hand. Follow the directions for the volar-based splint to create the individual finger troughs. Make sure all edges on the pre-cut MP finger and thumb openings are rolled back sufficiently so as to avoid putting pressure on the dorsum of the MP joint itself. Smooth all edges as necessary and attach a forearm strap.

## REFERENCES

This pattern is from the Rehabilitation Division, Smith & Nephew Inc. catalog. This splint design is courtesy of Bronwyn Keller, OTR.

Note: For an in-depth discussion on the efficacy of volar versus dorsal splints for muscle tone reduction, see Appendix C.

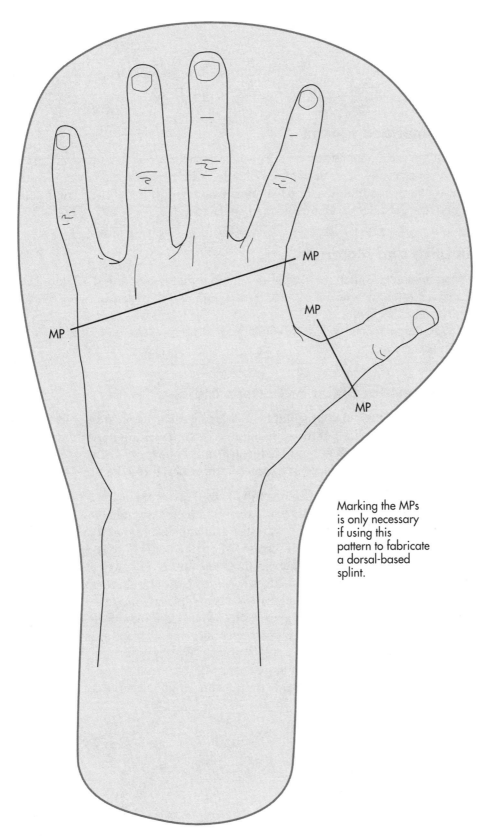

Marking the MPs
is only necessary
if using this
pattern to fabricate
a dorsal-based
splint.

Figure **4.57** Volar Anti-Spasticity Splint

Copyright © 1998 by Therapy Skill Builders, a division of The Psychological Corporation/All rights reserved/
Laura Hogan and Tracey Uditsky, Pediatric Splinting/ISBN 0761615148/1-800-228-0752/This page is reproducible.

## Volar Elbow-Extension Splint

### Purpose

This splint is used to prevent further elbow flexion contracture or to improve current elbow-extension range.

### Recommended Patient

This splint is recommended for patients who have or are at risk for developing elbow-flexion contractures. This design may be selected for specific diagnoses including cerebral palsy, traumatic brain injury, brachial plexus injury, or other clinical conditions that place the patient at risk for an elbow-flexion contracture.

### Supplies and Materials

We recommend 1/8-inch thermoplastic material that is rigid but does not have a high degree of stretch. It does not need to have a high degree of conformability. Rubber materials such as Ezeform or Orthoplast work well. You will need self-adhesive hook Velcro and regular loop Velcro or Velfoam for strapping. Use moleskin or comfort padding as needed.

### Instructions for Splint or Pattern Making

Determine the length of your splint by measuring the distance from mid-forearm to mid-humerus. The width of the splint should be sufficient to drape around half the circumference of the arm at both the forearm and upper arm. Using these measurements, cut a rectangular-shaped piece of thermoplastic material (see Figure 4.60 on page 144).

Heat the material in water. Once it is fully heated, place the material on the volar surface of the patient's extremity while maintaining maximum elbow extension. Drape the material around the forearm and upper arm and ensure that there are no folds or unnecessary wrinkles at the elbow crease. Allow the material to cool fully with the elbow positioned in maximum to sub-maximum extension. Trim any excess length or width and flare both the proximal and distal edges away from the skin for comfort (Figure 4.58). Add strapping at the proximal and distal ends and place a single wide strap or two criss-cross straps at the elbow joint (Figure 4.59). If needed for comfort, line the splint with moleskin or padding. If you know you are going to pad the splint before fabrication, it is best to pre-pad with a closed-cell padding material *prior* to forming the splint on the patient's arm. This will provide a more customized fit, and it is easier to pad when the splint is flat than when it has already been formed and has curves.

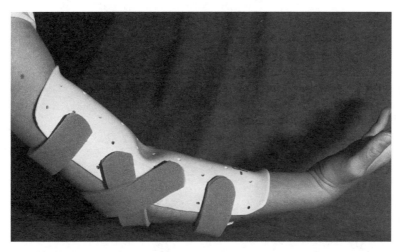

Figure **4.58**    Flare the edges away from the skin for comfort

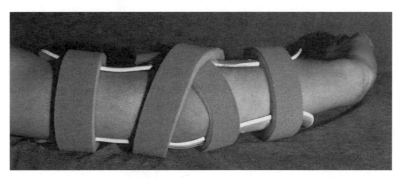

Figure **4.59**    An example of criss-cross strapping at the elbow joint

## REFERENCES

This basic splint design can be found in North Coast Medical and Rehabilitation Division, Smith & Nephew Inc. catalogs.

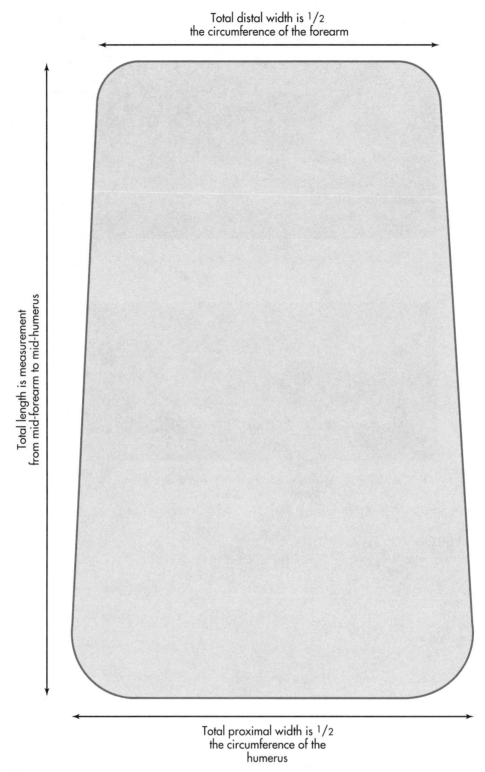

Total distal width is ¹/₂
the circumference of the forearm

Total length is measurement
from mid-forearm to mid-humerus

Total proximal width is ¹/₂
the circumference of the
humerus

Figure **4.60** Volar Elbow-Extension Splint

Copyright © 1998 by Therapy Skill Builders, a division of The Psychological Corporation/All rights reserved/
Laura Hogan and Tracey Uditsky, Pediatric Splinting/ISBN 0761615148/1-800-228-0752/This page is reproducible.

# Circumferential Elbow Splint

## Purpose

This splint is used to reduce or prevent contractures at the elbow. It may be used to maintain range of motion following casting or a surgical procedure. It also can be used to position the elbow in an extended position for function or may be used to extend the elbow during weight bearing.

## Recommended Patient

The circumferential elbow splint works nicely for patients with any amount of spasticity in the elbow flexors. It can be fabricated for single use or be used in a serial manner. Because this splint is made of a conforming elastic material that bends somewhat if the child has spasms, it is generally comfortable to wear. Because of the circumferential design, this splint is difficult for a child to remove independently. (It is actually difficult for an adult to don and doff independently.) This should be taken into consideration when selecting this type of splint for a patient.

## Supplies and Materials

You need 1/12-inch micro-perforated soft Orfit or a similar material. If you are working with a larger adolescent you may want to select a thicker material such as 1/8-inch Orfit Maxi Perforated. You will need three straps. A small amount of therapy putty to cover the olecranon or other bony prominences may be needed as well.

## Instructions for Splint or Pattern Making

Before making your pattern and cutting out the material you need to decide on a method of fabrication. You can fabricate this splint in a serial manner, enabling you to use the same material over and over as the child's range increases, or you can fabricate it for single use, requiring subsequent splints to be made with new pieces of material. As it is difficult to position the elbow while you are fabricating the splint, we recommend that you ask for help if you can.

The overall shape of the splint for both methods is similar to that shown in Figure 4.64 on page 148. The patterns are quick and easy to make. You will need four measurements: the length of the arm from halfway up the humerus to halfway down the forearm (A), the circumference of the forearm at the distal end of the splint (B), the circumference of the elbow at the crease (C), and the circumference of the humerus at the proximal end of the splint (D).

## Directions for Serial-Use Splint

Take the circumferential measurements and add 2 to 2 1/2 inches to each. Draw a pattern. Lay one edge of material on the most lateral aspect of the volar surface. Wrap the material over the volar surface (Figure 4.61). Place a wet paper towel over the volar surface of the splint. (This paper towel is important. It will keep the material from sticking to itself.) Continue to wrap the material around the elbow. Overlap the material onto itself (Figure 4.62). Allow the material to set and then remove the paper towel. Because a thin elastic material was used to make this splint, the cooled splint can be pulled

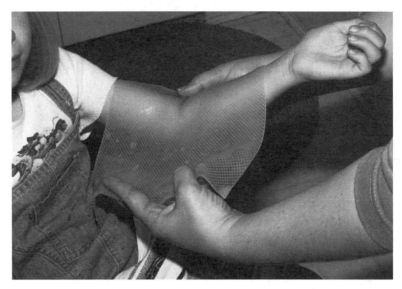

Figure **4.61** Starting position for the splint designed for serial use

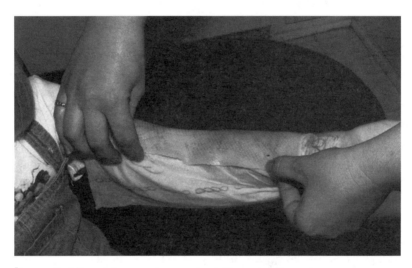

Figure **4.62** In the serial use splint, the material overlaps onto itself and a paper towel is used to keep the material from sticking to itself

open wide, enabling you to remove it from the patient's arm. As mentioned previously, if the splint is large or the child has severe spasticity, it may be difficult to get the splint on and off. Trim the overlapping portion of the splint until it lies on the volar surface only. You need only a few inches to overlap. Secure with three small straps. (Remember to select a strap that can be removed, as you are planning to refabricate this splint.)

## Directions for a Single-Use Splint

Take the circumferential measurements and add 1 to 1 1/2 inches to each. Draw a pattern. With the arm positioned as desired and prominences padded if needed, place the heated material on the volar surface and pinch the edges together on the lateral border of the

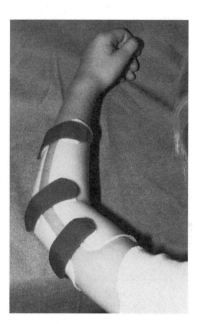

Figure **4.63** Completed single use splint demonstrating a ½-inch to 1-inch gap on the lateral border of the arm

arm. Once the sides are pinched, you can smooth the material and continue to position the arm as desired. When the material is almost cool, unsnap the sides. Trim the sides leaving about a 1/2-inch to 1-inch space between them. Flare the proximal and distal ends and apply straps (Figure 4.63).

**Important Notes:** Some therapists like to pad elbow splints to increase the child's comfort. We feel padding may be unnecessary with this splint because its circumferential design spreads the pressure throughout the arm. It will be especially comfortable if you pre-padded the bony prominences with therapy putty and flared the proximal and distal edges so they do not dig into the muscle bellies. The idea behind this splint is to increase range through a slow, steady splinting program. Don't *crank* the arm to maximum range and splint. Instead, position the arm in its best possible alignment and splint in a submaximal range. Typically, when the splint results in 10° to 15° more extension at the elbow, it will need to be refabricated. If you want to pad, prepad your splinting material with a closed-cell pad before you heat it. Remember, if the splinting material is padded, it cannot "stick" to itself when you pinch the sides together as you do for the single-use splint. If you choose to pad the single-use splint, you will need assistance or something like a Chip Clip® to hold the flaps together as the material cools. After the material is cooled, the wet padding will take an additional hour or two to dry.

## REFERENCES

The design of this splint was shared with us by a North Coast Medical Supplies sales representative in 1994. If the goal of the circumferential elbow splint is to help the therapist position the child into weight bearing on an extended elbow during a treatment session, the Urias® air splints are latex-free inflatable splints that can be helpful. Although they can be a good way of extending the elbow during a treatment session, we do not recommend that the air splints be used to prevent contractures or to increase range of motion. They have the potential to impede circulation in the arm and should therefore be monitored closely during use. Urias splints come in pediatric sizes. They are available through Sammons Preston and AliMed Inc. They range in price from $21 to $28 plus shipping and handling.

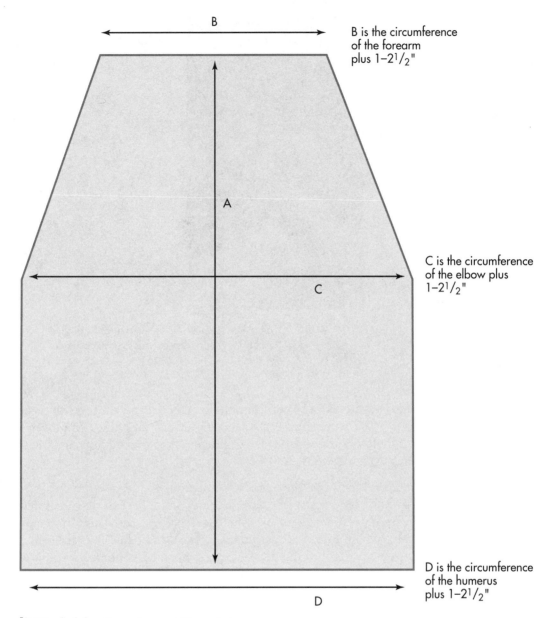

B is the circumference
of the forearm
plus 1–2$^1/_2$"

C is the circumference
of the elbow plus
1–2$^1/_2$"

D is the circumference
of the humerus
plus 1–2$^1/_2$"

Figure **4.64** Circumferential Elbow Splint

Copyright © 1998 by Therapy Skill Builders, a division of The Psychological Corporation/All rights reserved/
Laura Hogan and Tracey Uditsky, Pediatric Splinting/ISBN 0761615148/1-800-228-0752/This page is reproducible.

# Soft Elbow-Extension Splint

## Purpose

This splint is used to prevent further elbow-flexion contracture, to increase elbow-extension range, or to improve elbow crease hygiene and reduce tone.

## Recommended Patient

This splint design is recommended for patients who cannot tolerate a hard thermoplastic splint because of pain or skin integrity issues but are at risk for skin breakdown in the elbow crease or for further elbow-flexion contracture. Even though it is not a rigid splint design, this splint has been shown to increase joint range through its dynamic action. This design is used for both elbow- and knee-flexion contractures in the pediatric population.

## Supplies and Materials

You will need a piece of fire-retardant polyurethane foam that is 3 inches thick, of 1.8 to 2 pounds density, and with a firmness of 33 ILD (a measurement of firmness used for foam). The thickness and firmness of the foam depends on the age and size of the child and the degree of contracture. Additional supplies include terry cloth (enough to cover the foam), webbing, regular hook Velcro, regular loop Velcro, and a sewing machine.

## Instructions for Splint or Pattern Making

No pattern is used for this splint design. First, you must determine the dimensions of your splint by measuring the length and girth of your patient's extremity. The total length will be the distance from just proximal to the patient's wrist to the axilla of the patient's upper arm, minus 1 to 2 inches. The girth is determined by measuring the circumference of the extremity, both proximally and distally (Figure 4.65).

Using an electric knife or foam cutter, cut the polyurethane foam to the correct dimensions. Encase the foam in a terry cloth cover, sewing three edges and leaving the fourth edge open for easy insertion and removal of the foam. On the open edge, sew a strip of hook Velcro to one side and loop Velcro to the other to create a temporary Velcro closure the entire length of the terry-cloth cover. Next, sew three straps of 2-inch webbing material with Velcro fastenings to the terry-cloth cover. Position the central strap so that it fits directly over the elbow joint when worn. Attach the remaining two straps, one on either side of the central strap, to create a distal forearm and a proximal upper arm strap (Figure 4.65).

The foam splint should be wrapped circumferentially around the elbow. The edges should meet snugly but should not overlap. When placing the splint on the child, make sure the splint opening is not placed anteriorly or posteriorly, as this would allow the flexed elbow to escape. The seam should be placed on the medial or lateral border of the extremity. This splint is intended for wear at night but also could be worn during the day as appropriate.

Improvements in range are more likely to be noted with younger populations. Over time, the foam softens, and the splint must be refabricated at regular intervals. The terry-cloth cover is used because it ensures equal distribution of pressure, is comfortable, absorbs perspiration, and can be removed for regular washing.

This splint can be modified by varying the foam thickness (2-inch foam is often preferred for smaller children) and by varying the density. We also have used orthopedic felt to fabricate this same design on infants when the foam was too bulky and caused excessive upper-extremity abduction.

## REFERENCES

Anderson, J.P., Snow, B., Dorey, F.J., & Kabo, J.M. (1988). Efficacy of soft splints in reducing knee-flexion contractures. *Developmental Medicine and Child Neurology, 30,* 502–508.

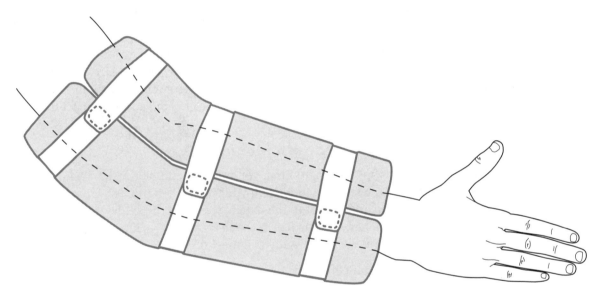

Figure **4.65**   Soft Elbow-Extension Splint

## Dynamic Elbow-Flexion Splint

### Purpose

This splint is used to facilitate elbow flexion without inhibiting elbow extension.

### Recommended Patient

This splint design originally was intended for use with the severe elbow-extension contractures that can result from the effects of arthrogryposis. We have found that the use of this splint can also be expanded to brachial plexus injuries or any other clinical condition where the elbow extension is secondary to an orthopedic, rather than a neurological, cause. The goal of the splint is to stretch the elbow progressively and facilitate elbow flexion. The splint can be worn during the day as it does not interfere with functional activities because it does not prevent the child from using active elbow extension. This splint can be used with children who do not demonstrate any *active* elbow flexion. However, the best results occur when the child has at least some *passive* elbow flexion.

### Supplies and Materials

You will need a rubber or plastic-rubber thermoplastic material to fabricate the chest harness. This material does not need to be highly conforming or rigid. Recommended materials include Synergy, Orthoplast, or Polyflex II. In addition, you will need to fabricate a wrist cock-up splint with thumb hole out of an elastic, rubber, or plastic-rubber material. Your material choice for the cock-up splint will depend on the amount of conformability required for your patient's needs. For strapping, you will need self-adhesive hook Velcro and either regular loop Velcro, Velfoam, or another appropriate strapping material of your choice. For the traction component, you will need latex tubing or Thera-Band® Tubing™.

### Instructions for Splint or Pattern Making

**To make the harness:** Using a cloth measuring tape, measure the distance from the child's anterior-superior iliac spine, over the shoulder, and then down to the iliac crest of the pelvis. Cut two strips of material 1 1/2 inches wide by the determined length (the distance from anterior iliac spine to posterior iliac crest). Heat and mold these strips, draping them over the child's shoulders and allowing them to grossly conform to the trunk from the anterior-superior iliac spine to the iliac crest. You may need to roll the edges slightly at the shoulder to allow for full active shoulder motion (Figure 4.66). To keep the harness stationary and prevent it from slipping off the shoulders, cut a wide strip of thermoplastic material and bond it (with heat, glue, or rivets) to both the left and right anterior harness straps so that it runs horizontally across the chest (Figure 4.67). Attach self-adhesive hook Velcro to the distal-most portion of both the left and right harness. You will need to attach the hook Velcro to both the anterior and posterior surfaces. Cut a long strip of regular loop Velcro. This will be used when the child is wearing the harness to secure it to the child's trunk (Figure 4.68).

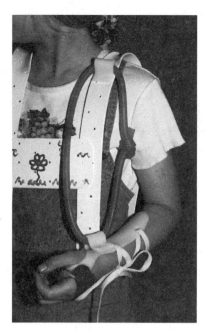

Figure **4.66** Slightly roll the edges at the shoulder to allow full movement

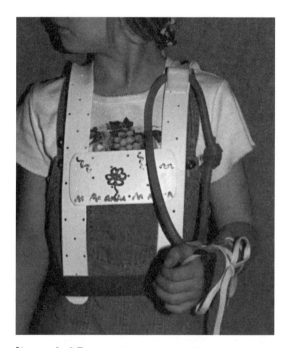

Figure **4.67** An anterior view of the harness

**To make the hand splints:** Follow the pattern and fabrication instructions for the volar cock-up with thumb hole splint. You may need to make unilateral or bilateral splints depending on the child's diagnosis. If the child has bilateral involvement, such as with arthrogryposis, bilateral splints may be indicated. Keep in mind, however, that in order for the child with arthrogryposis to achieve maximum function, it may be preferable to facilitate elbow flexion only in one extremity (for feeding and upper extremity dressing),

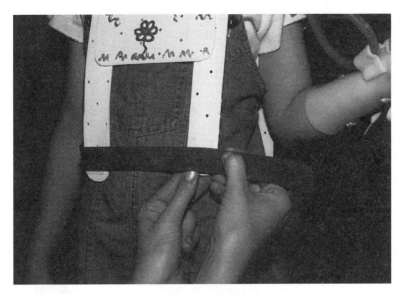

Figure **4.68** Loop Velcro is used to secure the harness to the child's trunk

while allowing the opposite extremity to remain contracted in extension (for toileting and perineal care).

The diagnoses that we have used this splint for include brachial plexus injury and arthrogryposis. Therefore, a volar wrist cock-up splint was an appropriate choice for the hand-splint portion of this splint design. If the wrist is not flexed and a cock-up splint is therefore not appropriate, you should not fabricate one. Other options for the hand-splint portion include a neoprene thumb-abduction splint, a thumb spica, or any other splint that you have determined to be appropriate. Whatever you select to fabricate, you will need to find a way to attach a loop (refer to the following directions). Loops made out of materials other than thermoplastics will work, but we do not recommend making a loop out of a material that stretches. It will interfere with the tension of the tubing. The only dynamic force should be coming from the tubing and not from the "give" of the loop. For this reason, we recommend you select a material such as webbing and avoid materials such as neoprene.

**To make the traction component:** To provide the traction component, you must thread a piece of stretchable tubing between the shoulder harness and the hand splint(s). First, bond a small thermoplastic loop to the harness above the clavicle and a second loop to the splint above the radial styloid. Make sure that the loops have a large enough opening to allow the tubing to be threaded through. Thread the tubing through the splint loop, through the shoulder harness loop, and tie a knot in the tubing (Figure 4.69). The amount of resting elbow flexion is determined by the amount of tension you create with the tubing. For more tension, tighten your tubing and for less tension, loosen the tubing. As the child ambulates, constant proprioceptive feedback is provided as a subtle "bouncing" motion is created through the dynamic force of the tubing. The loops through which the tube is inserted must withstand a lot of force and should be securely attached.

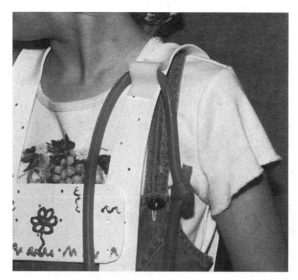

Figure **4.69** Tubing is threaded through the harness loop and then secured with a knot

## REFERENCES

Kamil, N.I., & Correia, A.M. (1990). A dynamic elbow flexion splint for an infant with arthrogryposis. *The American Journal of Occupational Therapy, 44,*(5) 460–461.

# Mitt Weight-Bearing Splint

## Purpose

This splint is used to simulate normal patterns of upper-extremity positioning during weight-bearing activities. It is designed to maintain the wrist in extension and prevent the hand from fisting so that weight bearing can occur through an open hand. This splint is intended to be a therapeutic tool and therefore is worn during therapy activities only.

## Recommended Patient

This splint design is intended for clients with increased muscle tone or other clinical conditions that create difficulty with weight bearing in the upper extremity with the hand in an open position. It is appropriate for patients with mildly increased tone as is seen in some cases of cerebral palsy or traumatic brain injury. It also is appropriate for children with brachial plexus injury (Erb's palsy) who tend to hold their wrist in flexion and will even attempt to weight bear on the dorsum of their hand.

## Supplies and Materials

Select a thermoplastic material that has a low degree of stretch. It does not need good conformability but should be at least moderately rigid to sustain the weight bearing. Recommended materials include rubbers and plastic-rubbers. In addition to the thermoplastic, you will need self-adhesive hook Velcro and regular loop Velcro or Velfoam for strapping.

## Instructions for Splint or Pattern Making

On paper toweling, trace the patient's hand with the fingers extended and slightly abducted and the thumb maximally abducted. You do not need to trace each finger or the thumb in isolation (see Figure 4.71 on page 157). Mark the wrist joint on the radial and ulnar side. Leaving at least a 1-inch border, draw a mitten shape around the entire hand using a dotted line to mark the separation of the thumb from the index finger. At the wrist, make a horizontal band extending out from both the radial and ulnar sides to fit around the dorsum of the forearm.

The original design stops just proximal to the wrist joint but this pattern can be modified by extending the forearm portion two-thirds the length of the forearm as needed to disperse force for increased comfort. Trace the pattern onto the selected thermoplastic material, heat, and cut. Mold the splint on the volar surface of the patient's hand, allowing the PIPs and DIPs to be in slight flexion. This relieves the effects of tenodesis. Using a dowel or other cylindrical-shaped object, push the heated thermoplastic material up between the thumb and index finger (where you marked the dotted line), thus creating a ridge so the thumb is maintained in its own trough in maximal abduction and cannot adduct against the fingers. If you prefer, you can cut along the dotted line and mold an entirely separate trough for the thumb.

The wrist should be in 50° extension so that the majority of the weight-bearing takes place on the heel of the hand. The horizontal wristband should wrap around to the dorsal surface of the forearm, just proximal to the wrist joint. If needed, flare this proximal portion away from the wrist to prevent rubbing and pressure. A Velcro strap can be attached to either end of the wristband for improved closure (Figure 4.70). If excessive

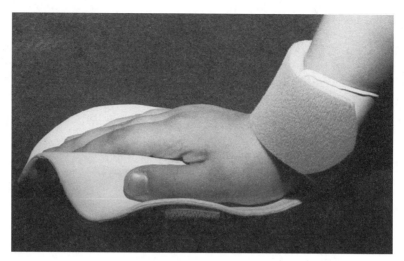

Figure **4.70** A wide Velcro or Beta Pile strap will secure the wrist portion

finger flexion occurs, try adding a Velcro or Velfoam criss-cross strap over the dorsum of the fingers to maintain extension. If this is not sufficient and the fingers continue to pull into flexion or even pull into a total fisted position, consider making the clamshell weight-bearing splint (see the next splint).

## REFERENCES

This splint design was adapted from Lindholm, L.A. (1986). Weight-bearing hand splint: A method for managing upper extremity spasticity. *Physical Therapy Forum with Occupational Therapy Forum*, 5(3), 1–4.

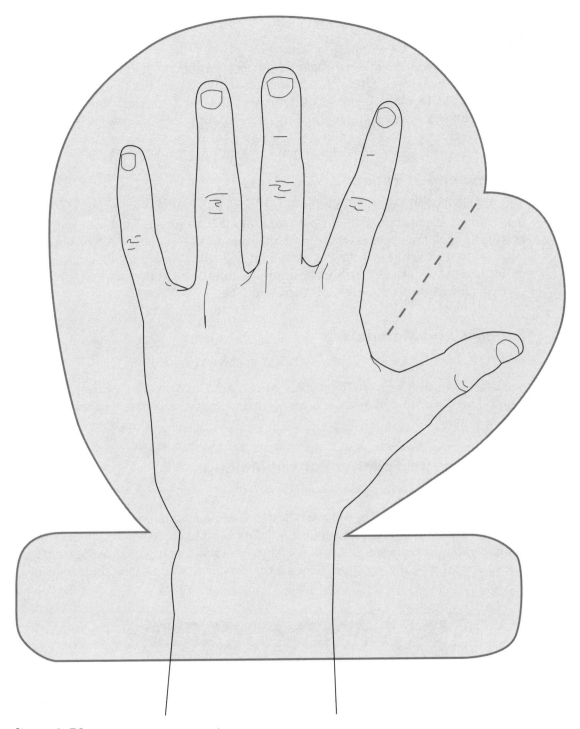

Figure **4.71** Mitt Weight-Bearing Splint

Copyright © 1998 by Therapy Skill Builders, a division of The Psychological Corporation/All rights reserved/
Laura Hogan and Tracey Uditsky, Pediatric Splinting/ISBN 0761615148/1-800-228-0752/This page is reproducible.

## Clamshell Weight-Bearing Splint

### Purpose

This splint is used to maintain the hand in an open position with the thumb and fingers in abduction and extension, and the wrist in extension during upper-extremity weight bearing. In addition, the splint facilitates palmar arch development. This splint is intended to be a therapeutic tool and therefore is worn during therapy activities only (Figure 4.76).

### Recommended Patient

The clamshell weight-bearing splint is recommended for patients with moderately increased muscle tone or other clinical conditions that create difficulty with weight-bearing through the upper extremity with the hand in an open position. The dorsal "shell" prevents the fingers from flexing and pulling out of the splint, which is a common problem noted with traditional weight-bearing splints (such as the mitt design) that are used on the hand with more severely increased tone.

### Supplies and Materials

**Base:** Use either 1/8-inch Aquaplast or Adapt-It Thermoplastic Pellets.

**Shell:** Use 1/16-inch perforated Aquaplast or 1/12-inch micro-perforated soft Orfit. You also will need a mound of medium firmness therapy putty, self-adhesive hook Velcro, and regular loop Velcro.

### Instructions for Splint or Pattern Making

No pattern is used to fabricate this splint.

**Directions for the base using a thermoplastic:** Using medium firmness therapy putty, make a mound that is large enough for the child's hand to depress into and leave an imprint without any fingers going off the edge. Heat a square of Aquaplast in hot water. The square must be slightly larger than the patient's hand while it is positioned in an

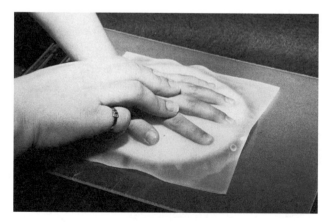

Figure **4.72**  The child's weight bears into a mound of therapy putty to create a customized base

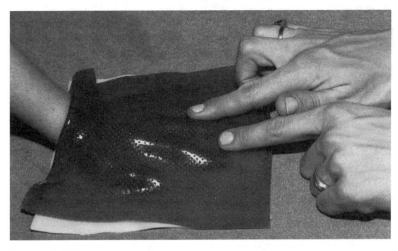

Figure **4.73** When making the dorsal shell, allow the material to drape down between each finger. Flare the material away from the wrist to allow extension

extended and abducted position. When it is heated, place the warm Aquaplast on top of the mounded therapy putty. Quickly position the child's hand in wrist extension and thumb and finger extension and abduction. Firmly place the hand onto the Aquaplast, pushing it into the mound to create a three-dimensional hand imprint (Figure 4.72). The putty with hot Aquaplast over it should ooze up slightly between each finger as well as between the thumb and index finger. Once a deep imprint has been created, remove the patient's hand and quickly cool down the Aquaplast (while it is still on top of the putty mound). Once it is completely cooled, pull the thermoplastic material off the putty. Trim the edges by rounding all corners, making sure not to trim off any of the hand imprint.

**Directions for the base using Adapt-It Thermoplastic Pellets:** Place a large handful of pellets into hot water. You will need enough pellets to create a mound large enough for the child's hand to depress into and leave an imprint without any fingers going off the edge. Make sure that while the pellets are heating they stay generally clumped together in the hot water. You can use a spatula to push any strays towards the mass. Once they are fully heated, the pellets will turn clear and you can remove them from the water using the spatula. Quickly knead the pellets together to form a uniform mass and place the mound onto a hard surface such as a clipboard. Quickly position the child's hand in wrist and finger extension and thumb and finger abduction. Push the hand into the mound creating a three-dimensional hand imprint. The mound of pellets should ooze up slightly between each finger and between the thumb and index finger. Once an imprint has been established, immerse the pellet mound in cold tap water with the child's hand still in place to cool it completely. Once the mound has cooled, remove the child's hand.

**Directions for the dorsal shell:** Cut a square of thin thermoplastic material (1/12 or 1/16 inch) that is large enough to cover the entire dorsum of the hand, extend slightly past the fingertips, and extend about 1-inch proximal to the wrist joint. Heat the thermoplastic material in hot water. While the material is heating, place the child's hand into the cooled base splint and have him or her weight bear into it with the wrist in maximum extension.

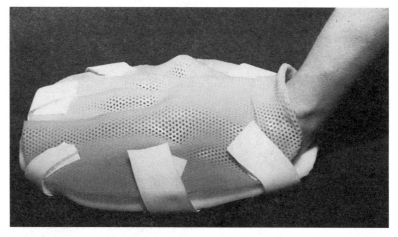

Figure **4.74** Regular loop and self-adhesive hook Velcro are used to attach the base to the shell

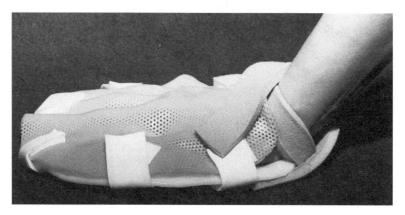

Figure **4.75** An alternative criss-cross wrist strap may provide more secure attachment

Place the heated dorsal piece over the child's hand and help the material drape down between each finger so a well-contoured dorsal shell is created. Make sure to maintain the wrist in extension and flare or fold the edge away from the dorsum of the wrist for comfort (Figure 4.73).

Quickly cool the shell while it is still on the child's hand. Once it has completely cooled, remove the shell and trim the edges by rounding off the corners to match the size of the base. To attach the base and dorsal shell together, place several short Velcro straps around the entire circumference of the splint. To do this, attach self-adhesive hook Velcro squares to both the base and the dorsal shell, with a short loop strap attaching the two pieces (Figure 4.74). If you believe your patient is at risk for pulling out of the splint you can use an alternative criss-cross strap at the wrist for more secure placement. This strap is used in addition to the circumference straps (Figure 4.75).

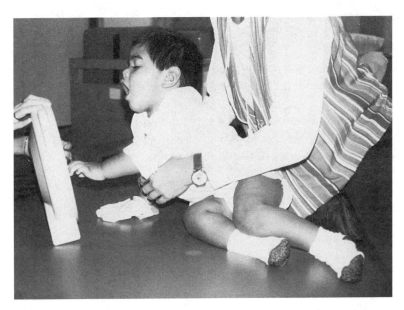

Figure **4.76**    A child uses the clamshell weight-bearing splint
during therapy

## REFERENCES

This splint design was taught to the authors by a North Coast Medical product representative.

## Palmar Hygiene Splint

### Purpose

This splint is used to open the palm of the hand and position it to promote elongation of the soft palmar tissue. It can be used to allow air flow into the palm for hygiene reasons as well. This design allows the skin in the hand to remain dry, promotes healing, and reduces odor caused by constant, moisture and skin breakdown. In order to inhibit the moisture and resulting skin breakdown caused by a constantly fisted hand, this splint should be worn the majority of the day and can be used at night as necessary.

### Recommended Patient

This splint is intended to be used on the severely involved patient who has no volitional ability to open the hand. When a patient has had a long-standing position of a tightly fisted hand that results in secondary moisture, odor, and skin integrity conditions, this splint can be highly effective. Its intent is not to gain maximum range of motion or even to position in optimum alignment, but initially is used just to address the hygiene problem. Even though improving range of motion is not the primary goal, when the splint is formed correctly it will directly influence the soft tissue in the palm. Improvements in range of motion caused by soft-tissue constrictions will result.

### Supplies and Materials

This splint is intended to be a serial static design. Therefore you must select an elastic material that has 100% memory. In addition, you need a material that is highly perforated to allow air flow. Depending upon the spasticity your client presents, you may select a 3/32-inch or 1/8-inch material. Our best success has been with super-perforated (42% perforations) Aquaplast, 1/8-inch thick. In addition, you will need self-adhesive hook Velcro and regular loop Velcro or Velfoam for a hand strap. Aquaplast Ultra Thin Edging Material may be used to finish the edges if desired.

### Instructions for Splint or Pattern Making

Using paper toweling, trace the patient's hand with the thumb slightly abducted and the fingers adducted. You do not need to trace between each individual finger. Mark the anatomical points as shown on the pattern (see Figure 4.83 on page 166). Transfer your pattern onto the selected perforated material, heat, and cut. Before molding to the patient's hand, make sure you have cut along the dotted line to allow for the thumb abductor portion. Roll this thumb portion into a dowel shape and attach it lightly to itself (Figure 4.77).

Next, mold the splint to the patient's palm. Press the material firmly into the palm so it makes a strong contact and conforms well to the palmar arch and into any deep crevices created by over-exaggerated palmar creases. If the thumb is adducted into the palm, the goal is to get it out of the palm so you can conform the material to make a palmar arch support. However, you are not trying to achieve maximum thumb abduction or perfect alignment at this time. Allow the thumb to rest gently upon the dowel to prevent it from contacting the palm. If necessary, form an ulnar border on the finger pan to prevent ulnar drift. The MPs should be extended to the maximum range possible without compromising the critical palmar contact. Allow the splint to cool and then trim and

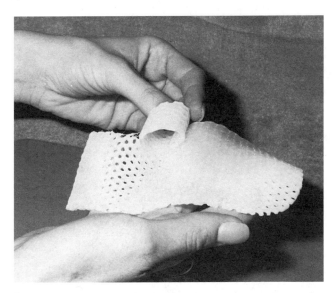

Figure **4.77**   Roll the thumb portion into a dowel shape

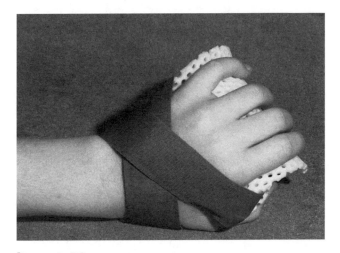

Figure **4.78**   Dorsal view of correct strapping

smooth any edges as needed. Remember that this is a hand-based splint and should not extend beyond the wrist. For strapping, add self-adhesive hook Velcro to the portion that covers the heel of the hand. Cut a long strap of regular loop Velcro or Velfoam. Feed the strap through the dowel opening of the thumb portion. Cross the free ends of the strap over each other to create a criss-cross strap over the dorsum of the hand (Figure 4.78). Then attach the free ends of the straps to either side of the heel of the hand (Figure 4.79).

This splint is categorized as a serial static design because it requires frequent modifications as the soft tissue constrictions are elongated. You will find that rapid changes in range of motion are made, and you may need to refabricate this splint several times. Because it is made with an elastic material, you can throw the entire splint back into hot water. The splint will flatten out into its original design and can then be remolded.

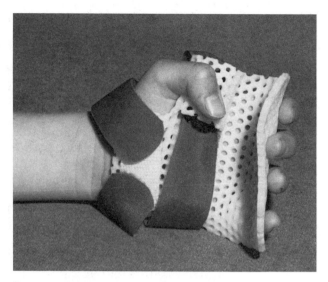

Figure **4.79** Volar view of correct strap placement

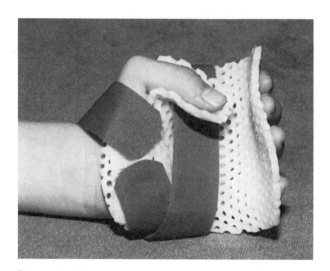

Figure **4.80** Volar view of the modified thumb cradle

Depending on the severity of the hand, you may be able to be more aggressive with the thumb positioning. A modification of this splint is to reverse the direction of the thumb dowel and form it into a thumb cradle (Figure 4.80). This can move progressively into more and more thumb abduction with each appropriate splint modification. When this splint design is selected for use with palmar hygiene problems (Figure 4.81), the key to its success is establishing firm contact with the palm by pressing the thermoplastic material aggressively against the patient's skin so soft-tissue stretching occurs. This firm contact is critical whether the cradle modification to the thumb is used or not (Figure 4.82).

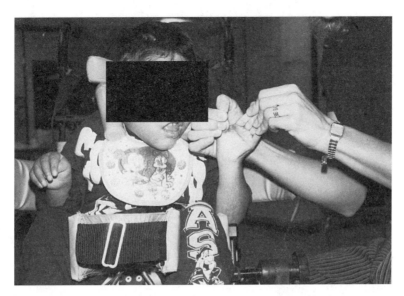

Figure **4.81** Tightly fisted hands lead to skin integrity and hygiene problems

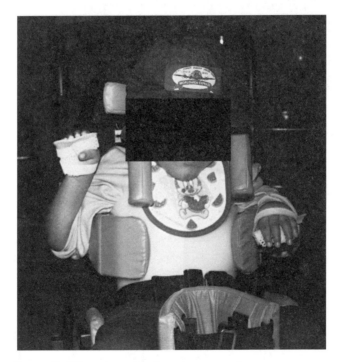

Figure **4.82** Bilateral palmar hygiene splints

## REFERENCES

The authors created this splint design.

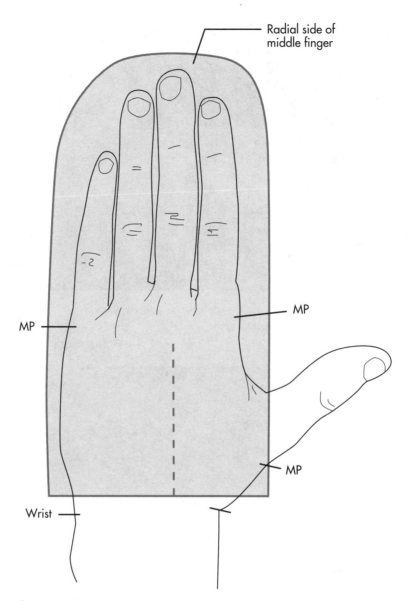

Radial side of middle finger

MP

MP

MP

Wrist

Figure **4.83** Palmar Hygiene Splint

Copyright © 1998 by Therapy Skill Builders, a division of The Psychological Corporation/All rights reserved/
Laura Hogan and Tracey Uditsky, Pediatric Splinting/ISBN 0761615148/1-800-228-0752/This page is reproducible.

# Palm-Protector Cone Splint

## Purpose

This splint is used on severely spastic or contracted hands to help open them and to protect them from the fingernails digging into the palm. It also can be used to improve hygiene or increase mobility of the tissues of the hand and fingers.

## Recommended Patient

Use these splints on patients with severe spasticity. If cone splints are made from a perforated material, they will allow air to reach the palm and enable damaged tissues to heal. Although their main purpose is to protect the palm, you also might consider using these splints as a beginning point of a splinting program for a hand that is so spastic or badly contracted that a wrist splint is impossible to apply.

## Supplies and Materials

Depending on the goal of your palm-protector cone splint you may want to select a rigid plastic material like Polyform or Kay Splint Basic I, or a highly perforated material like Aquaplast super-perforated. You can use a variety of thicknesses. Unless you are splinting with a perforated material to heal damaged tissues, you might want to pad the cone with moleskin or padding for added comfort. You will need one soft strap.

## Instructions for Splint or Pattern Making

Although there are several sources from which you can obtain an inexpensive palmar cone, you may prefer to fabricate your own, especially for your "youngest" patients or those you think will have rapid improvements in hygiene and may soon be ready to progress to a different type of splint. To make the cone, cut a piece of thermoplastic material in the shape of a curved wedge as shown in Figure 4.85 on page 169. You do not fabricate this splint on your patient's hand. (We sometimes cheat and fabricate the splint directly over an exercise cone from the clinic to get a good shape.) Make sure you don't have any sharp or uncomfortable edges where the palm or the fingers will be contacting the cone. Trim the cone at the top or bottom if the material does not line up well. Apply one strap through the middle of the cone across the dorsum of the hand (Figure 4.84). You can attach the strap permanently at one end inside the cone and have a second Velcro attachment at the other end.

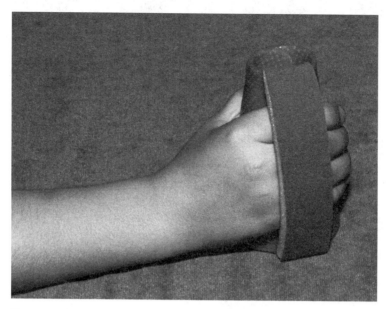

Figure **4.84** A finished splint with one soft strap over the dorsum of the hand

## REFERENCES

Prefabricated versions of this splint can be found in Rehabilitation Division, Smith & Nephew, Inc.; Sammons Preston; and AliMed Inc.

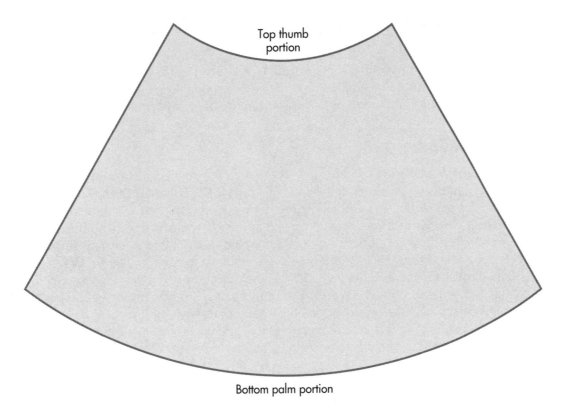

Figure **4.85** Palm-Protector Cone Splint

Copyright © 1998 by Therapy Skill Builders, a division of The Psychological Corporation/All rights reserved/
Laura Hogan and Tracey Uditsky, Pediatric Splinting/ISBN 0761615148/1-800-228-0752/This page is reproducible.

## Tri-Point Finger Splint

### Purpose

Use this splint to block finger PIP or thumb IP hyperextension while still allowing flexion. The splint design applies pressure at three points (one volar and two dorsal), creating a counterforce, that aligns the joint in the desired position.

### Recommended Patient

This splint design is intended for the patient with a swan neck deformity or other clinical conditions resulting in hyperextension at the PIP joint of the finger or the IP joint of the thumb. We have expanded the use of this design and now use it for children with athetosis who demonstrate hyperextension at the PIP joints when attempting to reach for and grasp an object. These children do not have a PIP hyperextension contracture at rest, but demonstrate this pattern only when attempting to actively grasp or release (i.e., during functional activities). This hyperextension pattern may be observed in all fingers or only one finger. Because the intent of the splint is to improve function, we usually splint only the index and middle fingers to allow for improved pincer and 3-jawed-chuck grasp patterns. It usually is not practical to splint all four fingers because the splints would be cumbersome and awkward for the patient to wear.

### Supplies and Materials

Select a solid thermoplastic that is thin (1/16-inch or 1/12-inch thick) and conforms well. We have had the best results with 1/16-inch Aquaplast. No strapping materials are needed.

### Instructions for Splint or Pattern Making

This splint design resembles a football goalpost (see Figure 4.88 on page 172). The "pole" must be the length of the measured distance from the mid-lateral border of the finger, under the volar PIP crease, to the mid-lateral border of the opposite side. The "uprights" come directly off the pole and must cross dorsally on either side of the PIP joint and wrap around the finger to the mid-lateral border on the other side (Figure 4.86). Cut a pattern out of paper toweling and size it on the patient. Once you have a customized, fitted pattern trace it onto your thermoplastic material and cut it out. You do not need to heat your material before cutting it because you can easily cut through a 1/16-inch thermo-plastic in its hardened form. Heat the material (it will only take about 20 seconds) and form it on your patient's finger. While forming, hold the patient's PIP joint in neutral or slight flexion. Make sure the material conforms snugly to all surfaces and that the pole is directly over the PIP crease on the volar surface to block any hyperextension. The joint should be free to flex and should not be covered dorsally by any portion of the splint.

If you are going to splint both the index and middle fingers, avoid having the uprights of the index finger touch the uprights of the middle finger. The splints should be worn so that the uprights face away from each other, allowing skin-to-skin contact between fingers (Figure 4.87). This way there will be less bulk between the patient's fingers and both splints can be worn comfortably at the same time.

Note: This splint design can be reversed to prevent a boutonniere deformity. When reversed, there are two volar points and one dorsal pressure, which block PIP flexion.

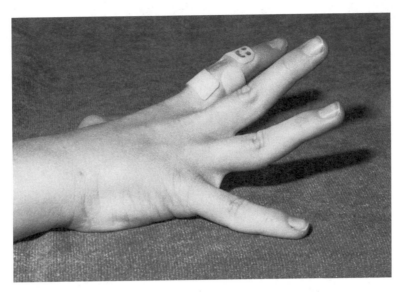

Figure **4.86**  Correct placement of the tri-point finger splint

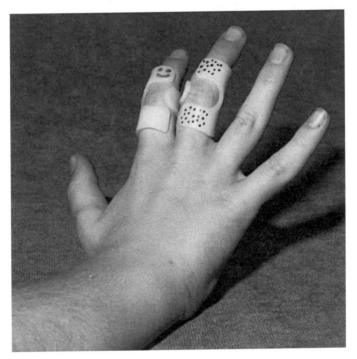

Figure **4.87**  Uprights should face away from each other if being worn on more than one finger

## REFERENCES

Melvin, J.L. (1983). *Rheumatic disease: occupational therapy and rehabilitation* (2nd edition). Philadelphia: F.A. Davis.

Murphy ring splints, which are commercially available prefabricated, stainless steel spring finger rings, can be purchased through North Coast Medical. These splints restrict hyperextension at the PIP joint(s) while still allowing active flexion. Adult sizes range from 2 (appropriate for pediatrics) to 13. Each splint is about $20 plus shipping and handling.

Ring splints or "figure-eight" splints also can be easily fabricated by wrapping Aquatubes around the finger. The tubes, available through Rehabilitation Division, Smith & Nephew Inc., come in varying widths. But even the narrow tubes tend to be bulky and in our experience often are discarded by patients.

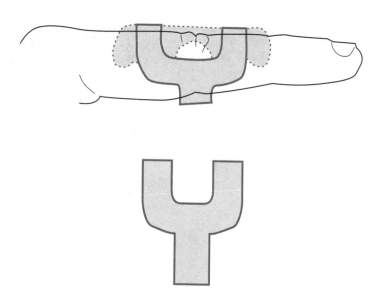

Figure **4.88** Tri-Point Finger Splint

Copyright © 1998 by Therapy Skill Builders, a division of The Psychological Corporation/All rights reserved/
Laura Hogan and Tracey Uditsky, Pediatric Splinting/ISBN 0761615148/1-800-228-0752/This page is reproducible.

# Suggested Reading

## 1. Anatomy

Moore, K. L. (1992). *Clinically oriented anatomy* (3rd ed.). Baltimore: Williams and Wilkins.

## 2. Normal Development and Fine Motor Skills

Bly, L. (1983). *The components of normal movement during the first year of life and abnormal motor development.*
This monograph may be obtained through:
The Neuro-developmental Treatment Association, Inc.
401 N. Michigan Ave.
Chicago, Illinois 60611-4267
(800)-869-9295

Alexander, R., Boehme, R., & Cupps, B. (1993). *Normal development of functional motor skills: The first year of life.* San Antonio, TX: Therapy Skill Builders.

Case-Smith, J., Pratt, P., & Allen, A.S. (eds.) (1996). *Occupational therapy for children* (3rd ed.). St. Louis, MO: C. V. Mosby.
Chapter 12 of this book is on the development of hand skills and contains some information on pediatric splinting as well.

Erhardt, R. (1994). *Developmental hand dysfunction: Theory, assessment, and treatment* (2nd ed.). San Antonio, TX: Therapy Skill Builders.

## 3. Splinting

Fess, E. E. & Phillips, C. A. (1987). *Hand splinting principles and methods* (2nd ed.). St. Louis, MO: C. V. Mosby.

Tenney, C. & Lisak, J. (1986). *Atlas of hand splinting*. Boston: Little, Brown and Company.

Keil, J. (1983). *Basic hand splinting techniques*. Boston: Little, Brown and Company.

Boheme, R. (1988). *Improving upper body control: An approach to assessment and treatment of tonal dysfunction*. San Antonio, TX: Therapy Skill Builders. (See Appendix A: Hill, S. *Current trends in upper-extremity splinting*.)

## 4. Myofascial Release

Barnes, J. F. (1991). *Pediatric myofascial release seminar manual*.
This manual may be obtained through:
Myofascial Release Treatment Centers
Rts. 30 & 252, Suite 1
10 S. Leopard Rd.
Paoli, PA 19301
(610) 644-0136

Manheiem, C. J. (1994). *The myofascial release manual* (2nd ed.). Thorofare, NJ: Slack, Inc.

## 5. Casting

Although this is a book about splinting, not casting, two resources for casting are included on the suggested reading list. Several of the goals of splinting are also achieved through casting and, in some select situations, casting may be an equally effective or even preferred method. Upper-extremity casting is beyond the scope of this book but for further discussion on its appropriate use, refer to the following resources.

Kelly, L. B. (1996). *Upper extremity casting. A practical guide*. San Antonio, TX: Therapy Skill Builders.

Boehme, R. (1988). *Improving upper body control: An approach to assessment and treatment of tonal dysfunction*. San Antonio, TX: Therapy Skill Builders. (See Appendix B: Yasukawa, A. & Hill, J. *Casting to improve upper-extremity function*.)

# Splinting Supply Resources

1. AliMed Inc.
   297 High Street
   Dedham, Massachusetts 02026-9135

   (800) 225-2610

   > Limited thermoplastics
   > Prefabricated splints
   > Strapping materials
   > Splinting supplies

2. Benik Corporation
   11871 Silverdale Way NW
   Silverdale, Washington 98383

   (800) 442-8910

   > Neoprene products
   > Prefabricated neoprene splints
   > Melco tape (neoprene heat sensitive tape)

3. Joe Cool Company
   2220 W. 200th S.
   Pingree, Idaho 83262

   (800) 233-3556

   > Prefabricated neoprene splints

4. North Coast Medical, Inc.
   187 Stauffer Boulevard
   San Jose, California 95125

   (800) 821-9319

Thermoplastic materials
Prefabricated splints
Neoprene
Strapping materials
Padding materials
Heat-activated Velcro (0143)
Iron-on neoprene tape (Melco tape)

5. Rehabilitation Division, Smith & Nephew, Inc.
One Quality Drive, P.O. Box 1005
Germantown, Wisconsin 53022

(800) 558-8633

Thermoplastic materials
Adapt-It Thermoplastic Pellets
Prefabricated splints
Neoprene
Strapping materials
Padding materials
Finger rivets

6. Rubatex Corporation
5223 Valley Park Drive
Roanoke, Virginia 24019

(800) 378-4081 or (800) 378-4093

Neoprene

7. Sammons Preston
P.O. Box 5071
Bolingbrook, Illinois 60440

(800) 323-5547

Thermoplastic materials
Prefabricated splints
Neoprene
Strapping materials
Padding materials
Rapid rivets
Permanent non-toxic colored markers

8. Velcro USA
P.O. Box 5218
Manchester, New Hampshire 03108

(800) 225-0180

Velcro products
Iron-on Velcro (0143)

# Efficacy of Volar Versus Dorsal Splints for Muscle Tone Reduction

Appendix **C**

The following is an article review:

McPherson, J., Kreimever, D., Aalderks, M., and Gallagher, T. (1982). A comparison of dorsal and volar resting-hand splints in the reduction of hypertonus. *American Journal of Occupational Therapy* 36(10), 664–670.

## Article Summary

The authors of this article looked at three previous articles whose research question was: "Does a static splint reduce hypertonus? If so, is a volar or dorsal splint better?" At the conclusion of their research review they conducted their own study with the same research question. The studies reviewed by the authors are summarized below:

1. Brennan (1959) studied 14 hemiplegic patients who wore splints 24 hours a day for a year. In his study abnormal muscle tone was abolished in all splinted joints. He suggested that splinting affected peripheral rather than central mechanisms, thereby altering the neuromuscular spindles' reaction to stretch.

2. Chariat (1968) splinted 10 patients with each type of splint and concluded that the pressure exerted by the volar splint resulted in increased muscle tone, the use of dorsal splints decreased muscle tone, and that constant splint-wearing could have adverse effects.

3. Snook (1979) concluded that a dorsal splint she designed reduced spasticity based on three case studies.

The authors of this article (1982) conducted their own study on 10 adults (ages 24 to 76, three who had cerebral palsy, all at least 1 year post-onset). Their research and study concluded the following:

1. Static splinting does reduce hypertonus.

2. Both types of splints reduce hypertonus.

3. Age plays a significant role in the amount of hypertonus that will be reduced. Those under 35 had a significantly greater decrease in muscle tone. Those over 65 did not demonstrate a significant tonal reduction.

**Interesting notes:**

The participants in the McPherson, J., et al., research wore the splints only 2 hours a day for 6 weeks. This would imply that splinting is a useful therapeutic procedure in a program designed for rehabilitation of the hand dominated by hypertonus. None of the studies clearly defines the effects of splint-wearing on the *reduction of contractures,* which is commonly the main objective of splinting a spastic hand.

# REFERENCES

Achenbach, C. L. (1993, March 8). A rule of thumb: Age-proofing static splints. *Occupational Therapy Forum*, 4–5.

Allen, K. D., Flegle, J. H., & Watson, T. S. (1992). A thermoplastic thumb post for the treatment of thumb sucking. *American Journal of Occupational Therapy, 46*(6), 552–554.

Anderson, J. P., Snow, B., Dorey, F. J., & Kabo, J. M. (1988). Efficacy of soft splints in reducing severe knee-flexion contractures. *Developmental Medicine and Child Neurology, 30,* 502–508.

Barnes, J. F. (1991). *Pediatric myofascial release* (pp. 5–6). Paoli, PA: Myofascial Release Seminars Workbook.

Bell, E., & Graham, H. K. (1995, September–October). A new material for splinting neonatal limb deformities. *Journal of Pediatric Orthopedics, 15,* 613–616.

Blair, E., Ballantyne, J., Horsman, S., & Chauvel, P. (1995). A study of a dynamic proximal stability splint in the management of children with cerebral palsy. *Developmental Medicine and Child Neurology, 37,* 544–554.

Blashy, M. R. M., & Fuchs, R. L. (1959). Orthokinetics: A new receptor facilitation method. *American Journal of Occupational Therapy, 13,* 226–234.

Bledsoe, S. (1994, September). To fabricate or not to fabricate: Splinting options. *Advance Rehabilitation,* 51–56.

Bly, L. (1983). *The components of normal movement during the first year of life and abnormal motor development.* Oak Park, IL: Neuro-Developmental Treatment Association.

Boehme, R. (1988). *Improving upper body control: An approach to assessment and treatment of tonal dysfunction.* San Antonio, TX: Therapy Skill Builders.

Bronski, B. (1995). Serial casting for the neurological patient. *Physical Disabilities Special Interest Section Newsletter, 18*(4), 4–8.

Case-Smith, J. (1995). Grasp, release, and bimanual skills in the first two years of life. In A. Henderson, & C. Pehoski (Eds.), *Hand function in the child: Foundations for remediation.* St. Louis, MO: Mosby-Year Book Inc.

Case-Smith, J., Allen, A. S., & Pratt, P. N. (1996). *Occupational therapy for children* (3rd Ed). St Louis, MO: Mosby.

Casey, C. A., & Kratz, E. J. (1988). Soft splinting with neoprene: The thumb abduction supinator splint. *American Journal of Occupational Therapy, 42*(6), 395–398.

Clemente, C. D. (Ed.). (1985). *Gray's Anatomy of the Human Body.* Philadelphia: Lea & Febiger.

Colangelo, C. A. (1993). Biomechanical frame of reference. In P. Kramer, & J. Hinojosa (Eds.). *Frames of reference for pediatric occupational therapy* (pp. 233–305). Baltimore: Williams & Wilkins.

Cruickshank, D. A., & O'Neill, D. L. (1990). Upper extremity inhibitive casting in a boy with spastic quadriplegia. *American Journal of Occupational Therapy, 44*(6), 552–555.

Eberhard, B. A., Sylvester, K. L., & Ansell, B. M. (1993). A comparative study of orthoplast cock-up splints versus ready-made Droitwich work splints in juvenile chronic arthritis. *Disability and Rehabilitation, 15*(1), 41–43.

Erhardt, R. P. (1994). *Developmental hand dysfunction theory, assessment and treatment.* San Antonio, TX: Therapy Skill Builders.

Exner, C. E., & Bonder, B. R. (1983). Comparative effects of three hand splints on the bilateral hand use, grasp, and arm-hand posture in hemiplegic children: A pilot study. *Occupational Therapy Journal of Research, 3,* 75–92.

Farber, S. D. (1982). *Neurorehabilitation: A multisensory approach.* Philadelphia: W.B. Saunders.

Fess, E. E., & Philips, C. A. (1987). *Hand splinting principles and methods.* St. Louis, MO: Mosby.

Flatt, A. E. (1972). Restoration of rheumatic finger joint function. III. *Journal of Bone and Joint Surgery, 54A,* 1317–1322.

Flowers, K. R., & LaStayo, P. (1994, July–September). Effect of total end range time on improving passive range of motion. *Journal of Hand Therapy,* 150–157.

Flowers, K. R., & Michlovitz, S. L. (1988). Assessment and management of loss of motion in orthopedic dysfunction. In *Postgraduate advances in physical therapy* (pp. 1–11). Alexandria, VA: American Physical Therapy Association.

Fox, S. (1991, April). What's new in splints? OTs are on the "cutting" edge. *Advance for Occupational Therapists,* 8–9.

Goodman, G., & Bazyk, S. (1990). The effects of a short thumb opponens splint on hand function in cerebral palsy: A single-subject study. *American Journal of Occupational Therapy, 45*(8), 726–731.

Hettinger, J. (1996). Pediatric splinting: Expect the unexpected. *OT Week, 10*(7), 12–13.

Hill, J. (1994). The effects of casting on upper extremity motor disorders after brain injury. *American Journal of Occupational Therapy, 48*(3), 219–224.

Hill, S. G. (1988). Current trends in upper-extremity splinting. In R. Boehme. *Improving upper body control: An approach to assessment and treatment of tonal dysfunction.* San Antonio, TX: Therapy Skill Builders.

Kamil, N. I., & Correia, A. M. (1990). A dynamic elbow flexion splint for an infant with arthrogryposis. *American Journal of Occupational Therapy, 44*(5), 460–461.

Kapit, W., & Elson, L. M. (1977). *The anatomy coloring book.* New York: Harper and Row.

Kerr, T. (1993, June). Today's market offers customized, job-specific splints. *Advance for Occupational Therapists, 10.*

Kiel, J. H. (1983). *Basic hand splinting: A pattern designing approach.* Boston: Little, Brown and Company.

King, T. (1982). Plaster splinting as a means of reducing elbow flexor spasticity: A case study. *American Journal of Occupational Therapy, 36*(10), 671–673.

Langlois, S., MacKinnon, J. R., & Pederson, L. (1989). Hand splints and cerebral spasticity: A review of the literature. *Canadian Journal of Occupational Therapy, 56*(3), 113–119.

LaStayo, P., & Jaffe, R. (1994, April–June). Assessment and management of shoulder stiffness: A biomechanical approach. *Journal of Hand Therapy,* 122–130.

Law, M., Cadman, D., Rosenbaum, P., Walter, S., Russell, D., & DeMatteo, C. (1991). Neurodevelopmental therapy and upper extremity inhibitive casting for children with cerebral palsy. *Developmental Medicine and Child Neurology, 33,* 379–387.

Lehmkuhl, L. D., & Smith, L. K. (1983). *Brunnstrom's clinical kinesiology.* Philadelphia: F.A. Davis.

Lind, W. R. (1992, January). Inhibitive weight bearing mitt/soft top design. *NDTA Network, 3.*

Lindholm, L. A. (1986). Weight-bearing hand splint: A method for managing upper extremity spasticity. *Physical Therapy Forum, 5*(3), 1–4.

MacKinnon, J., Sanderson, E., & Buchanan, J. (1975). The MacKinnon splint—a functional hand splint. *Canadian Journal of Occupational Therapy, 42*(4), 157–158.

Malick, M. H. (1982). *Manual on dynamic hand splinting with thermoplastic materials.* Pittsburgh: American Rehabilitation Educational Network.

Malick, M. H. (1972). *Manual on static hand splinting.* Pittsburgh, PA: American Rehabilitation Educational Network.

Marmer, L. (1993). The versatile art of plaster casting. *Advance for Occupational Therapists, 9*(23), 11.

Maunton, D. (1986). Materials used in orthotic fabrication. *Physical Disabilities Special Interest Section Newsletter, 9*(2), 2–3.

McClure, P. W., & Flowers, K. R. (1992). Treatment of limited shoulder motion using an elevation splint. *Physical Therapy, 72*(1), 57–62.

McClure, P. W., Blackburn, L. G., & Dusold, C. (1994). The use of splints in the treatment of joint stiffness: Biologic rationale and an algorithm for making clinical decisions. *Physical Therapy, 74*(12), 18–24.

McPherson, J. J. (1981). Objective evaluation of a splint designed to reduce hypertonicity. *American Journal of Occupational Therapy, 35*(2), 189–194.

McPherson, J., Kreimever, D., Aalderks, M., & Gallagher, T. (1982). A comparison of dorsal and volar resting hand splints in the reduction of hypertonus. *American Journal of Occupational Therapy, 36*(10), 664–670.

Melvin, J. L. (1983). *Rheumatic disease: Occupational therapy and rehabilitation* (2nd edition). Philadelphia: F. A. Davis.

Milder, N. (1991, April 8). Alternative splinting strategies for cognitively impaired patients. *Advance for Occupational Therapists, 11.*

Miura, T., Nakamura, R., & Tamura, Y. (1992). Long-standing extended dynamic splintage and release of an abnormal restraining structure in camptodactyly. *Journal of Hand Surgery, 17B,* 665–672.

Morehouse Marshall, N. A. (1989, June). Splints: One more twist. *OT Week, 4.*

Morris, S. E., & Klein, M. D. (1987). *Pre-feeding skills.* San Antonio, TX: Therapy Skill Builders.

Neuhaus, B. E., Ascher, E. R., Coullon, B. A., Donohue, M. V., Inbound, A., Glove, J. M., Goldberg, S. R., & Takai, V. L. (1981). A survey of rationales for and against hand splinting in hemiplegia. *American Journal of Occupational Therapy, 35*(2), 83–90.

Nolinske, T. (1986). Principles of upper limb orthotics. *Physical Disabilities Special Interest Section Newsletter, 9*(2), 1–6.

Osterhout, B. M. (1990). Postoperative splinting of the pediatric upper extremity. *Hand Clinics, 6*(4), 693–695.

Patterson, D., & Flanders, M. (1992, January). The pediatric arch orthosis: A combination splint for weight bearing and prehension. *NDTA Network,* 1–5.

Pearson, L. (1995, April). Hands on. *Team Rehab,* 21–27.

Reid, D. T. (1992). A survey of Canadian occupational therapists' use of hand splints for children with neuromuscular dysfunction. *Canadian Journal of Occupational Therapy, 59*(1), 16–27.

Reymann, J. (1985). The sof-splint. *Developmental Disabilities Special Interest Section Newsletter, 8*(2), 1–2.

Roholt, P. K. *Focus on splinting.* Centerville, OH: Clinical Specialty Education.

Schwanholt, C., Daugherty, M. B., Gaboury, L. T., & Warden, G. D. (1992). Splinting the pediatric palmar burn. *Journal of Burn Care and Rehabilitation, 14*(4), 460–464.

Sharpe, P. (1992). Comparative effects of bilateral hand splints and an elbow orthosis on stereotypic hand movements and toy play in two children with Rett syndrome. *American Journal of Occupational Therapy, 46*(2), 134–140.

Sharpe, P. A., & Ottenbacher, K. J. (1990). Use of an elbow restraint to improve finger-feeding skills in a child with Rett syndrome. *American Journal of Occupational Therapy, 44*(4), 328–332.

Smith, S. A. (1990, December 17). Splinting the severely involved hand. *Occupational Therapy Forum,* 9–11.

Smith, L. H., & Harris, S. R. (1985). Upper extremity inhibitive casting for a child with cerebral palsy. *Physical and Occupational Therapy in Pediatrics, 5*(1), 71–79.

Snook, J. H. (1979). Spasticity reduction splint. *American Journal of Occupational Therapy, 33,* 648–651.

Strickland, J. (1987). Anatomy and kinesiology of the hand. In E. E. Fess, & C. A. Philips. *Hand splinting principles and methods.* St. Louis, MO: Mosby.

Tatum, E. A. (1988, January). Serial casting for spastic posturing following neurologic injury. *Occupational Therapy Forum,* 12–14.

Tenney, C. G., & Lisak, J. M. (1986). *Atlas of hand splinting.* Boston: Little, Brown and Company.

Thompson-Rangel, T. (1991, September 20). The mystery of the serpentine splints. *Occupational Therapy Forum,* 4–6.

Tona, J. L., & Schneck, C. M. (1993). The efficacy of upper extremity inhibitive casting: A single subject pilot study. *American Journal of Occupational Therapy, 47*(10), 901–910.

Tuten, H., & Miedaner, J. (1989). Effect of hand splints on stereotypic hand behavior of girls with Rett syndrome: A replication study. *Physical Therapy, 69*(12), 1099–1103.

Wallen, M., & Mackay, S. (1995). An evaluation of the soft splint in the acute management of elbow hypertonicity. *Occupational Therapy Journal of Research, 15*(1), 3–13.

Yoshida, T., Daikoku, H., Yamamoto, H., Saitoh, S., & Saitoh, H. (1993, October–December). A flexible dorsal wrist splint. *Journal of Hand Therapy,* 323–325.

Yotsuyanagi, T., Yokoi, K., & Omizo, M. (1994). A simple and compressive splint for palmar skin grafting in young children with burns. *Burns, 20*(1), 55–57.